STEPHANIE TOURLES'S
Essential Oils
A BEGINNER'S GUIDE

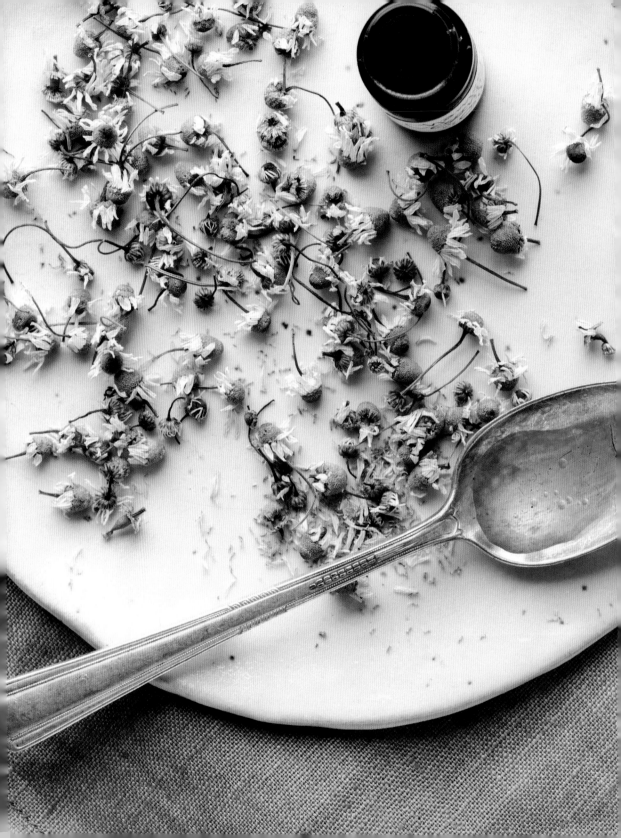

STEPHANIE TOURLES'S

Essential Oils

A BEGINNER'S GUIDE

Storey Publishing

The mission of Storey Publishing is to serve our customers by publishing practical information that encourages personal independence in harmony with the environment.

EDITED BY Deborah Balmuth and Lisa Hiley

ART DIRECTION AND BOOK DESIGN BY Michaela Jebb

TEXT PRODUCTION BY Jennifer Jepson Smith

INDEXED BY Nancy D. Wood

COVER PHOTOGRAPHS BY © BSIP/UIG/Getty Images, front (bottom) and spine; Mars Vilaubi, front (top right) and back; Michaela Jebb, front (top left); © Shutter Images/Daniel Watt, back (author)

INTERIOR PHOTOGRAPHY BY Mars Vilaubi

ADDITIONAL PHOTOGRAPHY BY © Alexandra Grablewski, i, v, viii, 4–5; © Amy_Lv/iStockphoto.com, 94; © Floortje/iStockphoto.com, 89; © Madeleine_Steinbach/iStockphoto.com, 77; © MC Yeung/iStockphoto .com, 133; Michaela Jebb, 188; © miguelangelortega/Getty Images, 75; © Nadezhda_Nesterova/iStockphoto .com, 198; © Paul Melling/Alamy Stock Photo, 52; © vikif/iStockphoto.com, 55; © Zoonar GmbH/Alamy Stock Photo, 175

PHOTO STYLING BY Raina Kattelson

This publication is intended to provide educational information for the reader on the covered subject. This book is not intended to replace professional medical advice or treatment. Read the instructions carefully and follow the safety precautions completely when making recipes.

The information in this book is true and complete to the best of our knowledge. All recommendations are made without guarantee on the part of the author or Storey Publishing. The author and publisher disclaim any liability in connection with the use of this information.

Storey books are available for special premium and promotional uses and for customized editions. For further information, please call 800-793-9396.

Storey Publishing
210 MASS MoCA Way
North Adams, MA 01247
storey.com

Printed in China by Toppan
Leefung Printing Ltd.
10 9 8 7 6 5 4 3 2 1

LIBRARY OF CONGRESS CATALOGING-IN-PUBLICATION DATA

Names: Tourles, Stephanie L., 1962– author.
Title: Stephanie Tourles's essential oils : a beginner's guide / Stephanie Tourles.
Other titles: Essential oils
Description: North Adams, MA : Storey Publishing, 2018. | Includes bibliographical references and index.
Identifiers: LCCN 2017061054 (print) | LCCN 2018004024 (ebook)
 | ISBN 9781612128757 (ebook) | ISBN 9781612128740 (pbk. : alk. paper)
Subjects: LCSH: Essences and essential oils—Therapeutic use. | Aromatherapy.
Classification: LCC RM666.A68 (ebook) | LCC RM666.A68 T68 2018 (print)
 | DDC 615.3/219—dc23
LC record available at https://lccn.loc.gov/2017061054

Contents

14 Additional Essentials

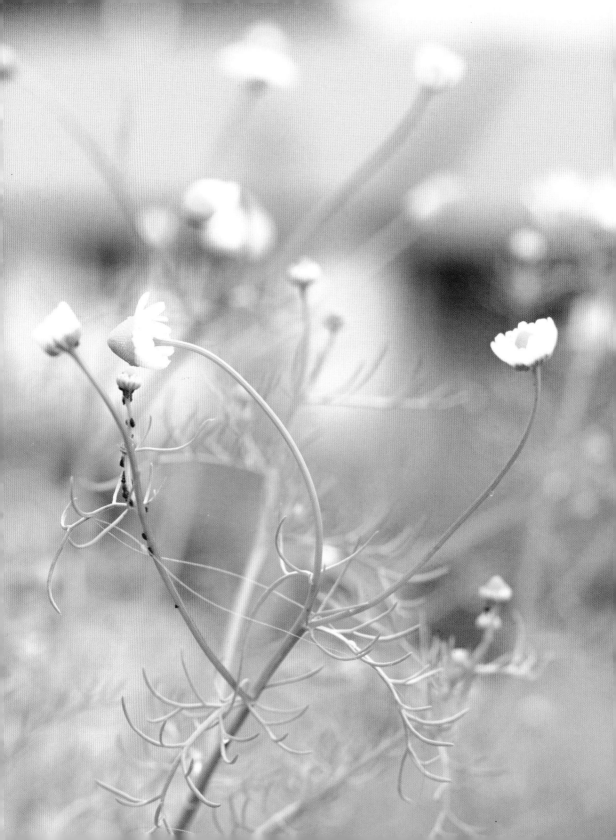

The Scent-sational World of Essential Oils

I can't tell you how many stories I've heard over the past two decades from folks who were disappointed with their initial foray into using essential oils. When they tried to treat their insomnia or speed the healing of a cut with a five-dollar bottle of poor quality or even synthetically adulterated lavender essential oil purchased from a corner drugstore or an online discount warehouse, nothing happened — or worse, they suffered a sneezing fit or developed an itchy rash. From one bad experience with "snake oil" instead of the therapeutically beneficial real deal, they chalked up essential oils as worthless hype!

That's so sad, because herbalism — using medicinal plants to support emotional, physical, and spiritual healing and well-being — is the oldest healing system on the planet. This traditional form of medicine, sometimes referred to as "the people's healing art," is enjoying an incredible resurgence in popularity worldwide, and for good reason — it is affordable and even more available and accessible than ever. Plus, it's safe!

Why am I talking about herbs in a book about essential oils? Well, because essential oils are potent, complex extracts or essences of herbs, spices, and other plants. They form the basis of the fragrant science of aromatherapy — the therapeutic application of pure, superior grade essential oils for physical and psychological well-being — which I consider a branch of herbalism. If you are interested in complementary medicine, especially the art and science of healing with plants, then the study of essential oils and aromatherapy should be explored, absorbed, and implemented in your daily life.

The achievements and advances in allopathic (conventional) medicine are amazing, but instead of always turning to a medical expert, it behooves you to develop the knowledge and skills to take more responsibility and control for your own and your family's health without totally relying on the medicines and policies of the mainstream medical system (which are viewed with varying degrees of skepticism by a growing number of folks).

Aromatherapy appeals on many levels, and its skyrocketing popularity might be growing more rapidly than other methods of natural healing, not just because its primary tools — essential oils — are readily accessible and available, but because those therapeutic oils smell so good, are effective and efficient, and come in convenient packages. These tiny bottles of concentrated aromatic plant essences can easily become nature's safe alternatives to the many synthetic chemicals that have invaded our lives and homes in the name of cleanliness, environmental enhancement, health, and well-being.

The initial impulse to learn about essential oils and aromatherapy is almost always instinctual, especially if you are drawn to plant medicine and all things fragrant, as I am. Books, courses, instructors, and even knowledgeable body workers such as estheticians, massage therapists, Reiki practitioners, and reflexologists, who often work intimately with essential oils, can

satisfy this educational impulse, yet learning about aromatherapy and using essential oils almost always turns into a vitalizing and dynamic process. It generally begins with a bit of experimentation.

Perhaps you decide to use an oil to revive your achy feet, relax after a long day, or ease a tension headache, and with a little luck there is some success, and you feel encouraged to continue. Thinking to yourself, "That was rather simple and quite pleasant, what other common ailments can I learn to treat?" And so your journey begins. . . .

The magnetism of aromatherapy is undeniable and is attracting an increasing number of followers these days – including you, right? I'm assuming that you're intrigued by essential oils, desiring to learn more about these aromatic liquids; otherwise, why would you have picked up this book? Learning and living aromatically, understanding essential oils as a lifestyle and utilizing their power in a way that supports you and helps to experience balance, comfort, and health as often as you can, is what this book is about.

The content of this book is geared towards the "essential oil newbie" — the true beginner. It's unique in that it simply focuses on a core group of 25 common essential oils. Without diving into the details of essential oil chemistry, which can be explored in more specialized texts, I've explained the characteristics and therapeutic uses that I find most beneficial, as well as safety concerns of each oil accompanied by 100 easy-to-make recipes — incorporating only these 25 essential oils — that specifically pertain to basic home health-care and wellness/comfort enhancement. All of this is very useful and *practical* information for the beginner, which is the point of this book!

And I'll teach you how to be an educated, discerning consumer, so you can tell the difference between useless cut-rate essential oils and authentic top-quality ones.

It is my sincere pleasure to share the knowledge I have gained in over 30 years of study, experimentation, and practice using essential oils. Based on my experience with countless friends, neighbors, customers, clients, and students, plus much feedback from the readers of my natural skin and body care books, I feel confident in saying that one of the best ways to improve and enhance your health, well-being, and personal environment is through the natural pleasures offered by aromatherapy.

Life is short, so remember to take time to stop and smell the lavender, rosemary, peppermint, orange peel, and cloves . . . the aromatic realm is full of wonders, possibilities, therapy, and joy!

Stephanie

Mother Earth's medicine chest is full of healing herbs of incomparable worth.

ROBIN ROSE BENNET

1

Essential Oils 101

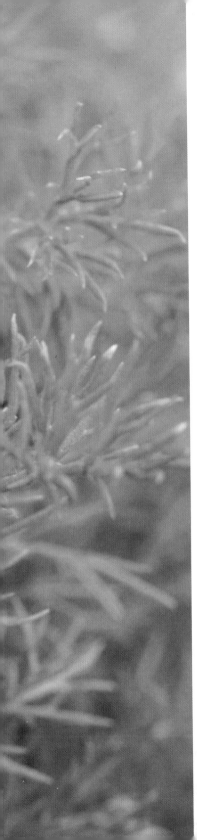

If you have ever enjoyed the heady scent of a rose blossom, the soft fragrance of lavender flowers, the cool pungency of a crushed peppermint leaf, the strong woody-resinous-herbaceous notes emanating from chopped rosemary, the crisp "Christmasy" scent that clings to your fingers after you put up a holiday balsam fir, the sweet and spicy fragrance of cinnamon and cloves wafting through the kitchen while an apple pie bakes in the oven, or the bright essence that oozes from an orange or grapefruit when you remove its rind, then you've experienced the aromatic qualities of essential oils. These fragrances appeal on so many levels, and oh, aren't they simply wonderful?

But what exactly are you smelling? Essential oils exist in plants as miniscule droplets that are stored in tiny secretory glands, glandular hairs, cavities, veins, and ducts of various plant parts. They are the "essence" (or even the "soul" or "spirit," as some aromatherapists like to say) of that particular plant, responsible for giving the plant its unique scent and chemical makeup.

Aromatic plants contain from 0.005 to 10 percent essential oil, with the average amount being 1 to 2 percent. With citrus fruits, the uplifting, refreshing essential oil squirts out in such profusion that it's easy to collect, but not all plants contain essential oil in such quantity. It takes 40 to 60 rosebuds, for example, to produce a single drop of rose otto essential oil — that's 600 pounds of rose petals for a single ounce of essential oil! It takes nearly eight million jasmine blossoms, hand-picked on the day the flowers open, to produce just over 2 pounds of superior essential oil. For tart-sweet lemon balm, one of the rarest essential oils, upward of 3 tons of fresh leaves and flowering tops are distilled to make 1 pound of essential oil. Not surprisingly, rose, jasmine, and lemon balm are three of the most expensive essential oils on the market.

Thankfully, not all plant materials are that stingy with their essential oil. One pound of essential oil can be extracted from approximately 250 pounds of rosemary leaves, 150 pounds of lavender buds, or 50 pounds of eucalyptus leaves, making the prices for these oils accordingly lower.

All-Time Favorites

Topping the list of the most popular essential oils are lavender, peppermint, lemon, sweet orange, and tea tree. This should come as no surprise, as they are some of the most affordable, versatile, and aromatically pleasing. Well, except for tea tree . . . its sharp medicinal aroma isn't so agreeable to the nose, that's for sure! But it more than makes up for this with its potent properties.

What's in an Essential Oil?

Essential oils are highly complex substances. Each one is a mosaic of hundreds — even thousands — of different chemicals. On average, an essential oil may contain anywhere from 20 to 400 identifiable constituents. Many oils contain even more, and it is the combination of all these components that give an essential oil its unique smell and impart its various properties, ranging from beneficial and therapeutic to toxic and hazardous.

In many ways, these oils are truly essential to the plants that produce them, being the secret weapons plants use to maintain their health on many

Essential oils have super-high-potency energy; use it wisely.

fronts: protecting themselves from diseases and pests, healing wounds, attracting both pollinators and herbivores that help the plant reproduce, and so on. These precious protective oils offer benefits for humans as well.

Chemically, essential oils have little in common with fixed oils, otherwise known as base or carrier oils, such as olive oil, sesame oil, and sweet almond oil. Essential oils do not contain fatty acids and are not prone to rancidity. Because of their molecular makeup they evaporate easily, hence their other common name, volatile oils. (The term *volatile* comes from the Latin root *volare*, which means "to fly.")

Most essential oils react with water much as fatty oils do, by floating to the top. They do, however, lend their scent to water and watery solutions (such as aloe vera juice or gel, witch hazel, and vinegar). They blend quite readily with base oils and other fats, and they dissolve to some degree in 80-proof ethyl alcohol, better in 100-proof alcohol, and completely in 190-proof pure ethyl alcohol, making them an ideal formulary ingredient.

Most essential oils at room temperature are a rather mobile liquid, being slightly thicker and less dense than water, but still effortlessly pourable. Essential oils can also be quite viscous (myrrh and frankincense), semi-solid (rose or cornmint), or even solid (such as orris root). Cold temperatures tend to thicken any oil, while heat makes them thinner.

Always keep in mind that essential oils are highly concentrated substances. Whether you're creating a jar of herb-infused oil or producing an herbal tincture, using essential oils is very different from using whole plant material. Only a small amount is necessary to induce a powerful benefit — we're talking *drops* versus teaspoons or even cups of fresh or dried herbs. Essential oils have super-high-potency energy; use it wisely.

What Can Essential Oils Do?

Essential oils offer myriad therapeutic properties that can be of much benefit to the body, mind, and spirit — you just have to know which ones to choose and how to use them properly to achieve the desired results. They have the ability to invigorate, refresh, calm, cleanse, cool, warm, boost immunity, relieve congestion, stimulate cognitive function, kill pathogenic microorganisms, reduce inflammation, increase circulation, act as a diuretic, relieve pain, minimize scar tissue formation — and that's only a partial listing! In my opinion, these plant-derived essences provide the most benefits for those who like to live in harmony with nature.

Essential oils are incredibly potent, so it's important to know what an oil does before you use it. All the essential oils discussed in this book are safe and gentle when used as directed.

The Making of an Essential Oil: Methods of Extraction

Essential oils are extracted from the plant by four different methods: steam distillation, expression, solvent extraction, and carbon dioxide gas extraction. Approximately 80 percent of essential oils are extracted by steam distillation.

Steam Distillation

This is the most common process for obtaining essential oils. During distillation, steam is forced under pressure through a vat of the plant material. The steam ruptures the oil reservoirs in the plant matter, releasing the volatile oil, which is captured and carried into a cooling unit, where it condenses. This condensed steam, called *distillate*, contains both the essential oil of the plant and a watery portion called *hydrosol*. The two fluids naturally separate, and both are collected and bottled.

The amount of essential oil yielded by steam distillation depends upon a number factors: distillation time, temperature, operating pressure, and the technique and expertise of the distiller. Most important is the type and quality of the plant material. A plant can contain more or less essential oil depending upon the time of harvest (the time of day / year), geography, climate, and soil conditions.

Expression

This method, also called *cold expression* or *scarification*, is used for extracting essential oil from citrus fruits, which contain large oil reservoirs in their outer peel. The peel is scarified or shredded and then mechanically pressed, resulting in an emulsion containing a blend of essential oil, juice, fruit particles, and water. The emulsion is either passed through a clarifying centrifuge or filtered. The essential oil floats to the top and is separated out.

Lemon and lime peel can also be steam-distilled, resulting in a particularly sweet-smelling, sweet-tasting oil that is frequently used for flavoring soft drinks and candy. These oils are considered inferior for aromatherapeutic use, as the heat from the steam alters their composition.

Solvent Extraction

This method of extraction uses solvents such as petroleum ether, hexane, toluene, butane, methane, and propane, and sometimes more toxic (carcinogenic) solvents such as acetone and benzene, to extract essential oil from plants whose structures are too delicate to withstand other methods, especially heat. Once the volatile oils, pigments, and waxes are extracted, the residual solvent is removed through evaporation under pressure. The result is a soft, sticky wax called a *concrete*, which is processed with ethyl alcohol and chilled. The solidified waxes are filtered out, leaving the volatile compounds diluted in the alcohol. In the final processing step, the alcohol is removed by vacuum distillation.

The resulting oil is referred to as an *absolute*. Due to the slight synthetic residue remaining in the end product, this type of essential oil is not considered of therapeutic grade, being deemed suitable solely for fragrance, such as in perfumes. Jasmine, rose, hyacinth, and mimosa are common absolutes. If an essential oil is an absolute, that fact will be indicated on the label.

Supercritical Carbon Dioxide (CO_2) Extraction

Sometimes you'll see the annotation "CO_2" after the name of an essential oil — for example, "frankincense CO_2." What does it mean? This relatively new method of extraction utilizes the "supercritical" state of CO_2, when it acts as both a gas and a liquid. The equipment required for this process is quite expensive, but the method yields a higher volume of essential oil, and the extraction is conducted under high pressure and relatively low heat without the use of steam or deleterious solvents that can degrade the quality of the essential oil. Carbon dioxide also extracts a wider range of molecules than does steam for a more complete and absolutely superior essential oil, without any chemical residue.

CO_2 extraction is most often used for the more expensive and oil-stingy plant materials, such as frankincense, myrrh, nutmeg, ginger, calendula blossom, and vanilla bean.

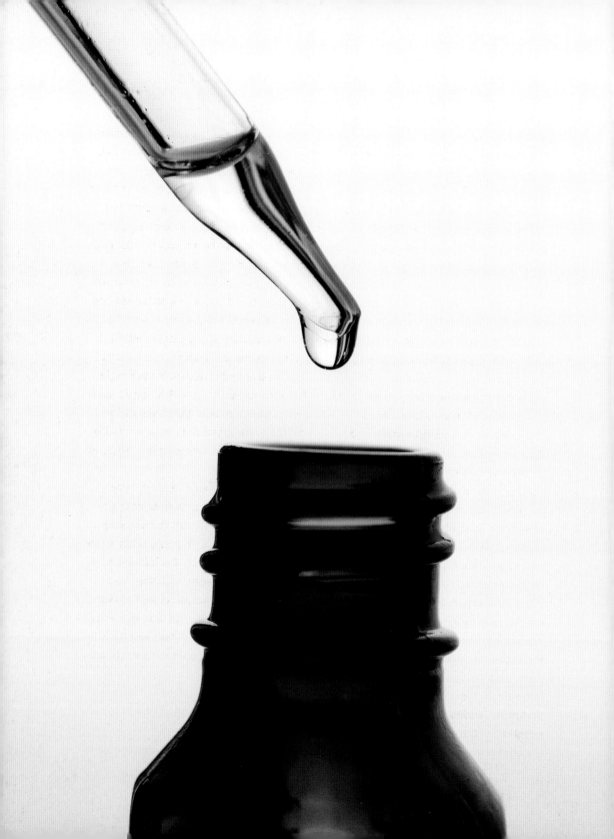

Sustainability

With the growth of an industry dependent on natural resources comes challenges, and the rapid boom in the sales of essential oils during the past decade has sparked concerns over sustainable sourcing. Securing a supply chain can definitely be challenging for an essential oil broker, retailer, or product manufacturer. Circumstances beyond the grower's or wild-harvester's control — climate conditions, pestilence or disease, labor availability, and civil unrest — all add layers of complexity and can lead to supply shortages.

I sometimes hear the argument that essential oils waste natural resources because they require too much plant material compared to other herb-based products. Well, I beg to differ. If highly concentrated essential oils are used properly, they can be both environmentally sustainable and economical. Granted, one drop of an essential oil does represent a lot of plant material, so use that precious drop while understanding and honoring its potency. Always remember, with aromatherapy, more is not better. Don't use 20 drops of peppermint in a revitalizing foot bath when 5 to 10 will suffice, nor 4 drops of lavender on a mosquito bite when 1 will do the job. Lower dilutions are not only economical but safer for the skin, too.

Certain essential oils such as Indian sandalwood, agarwood, and rosewood, though not discussed in this book, continue to be unsustainably produced from dwindling resources. Professional aromatherapy organizations and responsible aromatherapists do not support the continued use of essential oils from threatened species, especially when there are viable alternatives. Also worth watching are frankincense and myrrh, as they are in great demand but are collected from limited resources in areas of the world that tend to suffer from severe drought conditions. These five highly sought-after and valuable essential oils, in particular, are often subject to illegal poaching and trade, as they bring big bucks to the shady harvester.

It is your right and, I believe, your duty to ask your suppliers about their sustainability policies and where they obtain their oils. Consumer dollars speak loudly, and your purchases influence decisions that directly and indirectly impact our environment as well as economic and social policies. So I encourage you to ask questions and let your suppliers know that you are concerned about these vital issues.

2

Quality, Safety & Storage

The majority of essential oils are produced for the fragrance, food, and flavoring industries, not the therapeutic market, and the demand far exceeds the supply. Think about all the applications out there — cleaning and deodorizing products, laundry detergents, personal care products, cosmetics, perfumes, pharmaceuticals, and all manner of packaged foods and beverages. It's a long, long list.

Manufacturers have found that by mixing synthetics or other plant-sourced chemicals into their essential oils, or by producing totally synthetic oils, they can increase their supply and ensure that the desired scent/flavor never varies from a standardized norm, while keeping prices low. Adulterated and synthetic oils make up the bulk of inexpensive oils that are sold as 100 percent pure, natural essential oils. As far as I'm concerned, these oils have no therapeutic value whatsoever and should *never* be used on the body! Synthetic fragrances and flavors permeate our lives and are one of the most allergy-provoking substances we encounter.

Words of Wisdom

When you delve into the world of essential oils, you will surely study the works of Robert Tisserand, a chemist and essential oil consultant internationally recognized for his pioneering work in many aspects of aromatherapy. He truly understands both the chemistry and holistic nature of aromatic plants. This quote comes from his first book, *The Art of Aromatherapy*, which also happens to be the first book written in English (1977) on the subject of aromatherapy. It's a must-have addition to your essential oil library.

Essential oils are natural, organic substances. They are like milk in a mother's breast — a part of the plant, and yet a separate substance from the rest of the plant. As long as they are kept in proper conditions after distillation they will not lose their organic quality and hence their therapeutic value. Although the properties of essences are not always exactly the same as the plants they come from, essences do "represent" herbs to a large degree. The essence may not contain all the chemical constituents of the herb, but its vibration is similar, and it usually turns out to have the same properties. The essence is not the herb, but speaks for the herb, and has the same personality. The essence, as its name implies, is more concentrated and subtle than the herb; it acts on higher levels, and has a more pronounced emotional effect.

Why natural oils? Why not anything that smells nice whether it is natural or synthetic? The answer is simply that synthetic, or inorganic substances, do not contain any "life force"; they are not dynamic. Organic substances are those which are found in nature, like essential oils. "Organic" also means "structural," something which is "characterized by systematic co-ordination of parts in one whole." Nature has a structure which cannot be duplicated artificially. We can synthesize chemicals, but we cannot structure them to make something organic.

Quality Matters

All of the information presented in this book about the therapeutic qualities of essential oils pertains specifically to authentic, absolutely pure essential oils — not their cheap cousins masquerading as such.

Pure, high-quality essential oils have not been tampered with in any way. With their complexity and purity intact, they provide us with a pleasant, potent, effective, and convenient means to utilize the pharmacologically active constituents found in plants. We can use them to achieve results that their mass-produced, standardized, adulterated, restructured, synthetic, improperly distilled, or diluted namesakes can never hope to equal. Although the latter are considerably less expensive, they will not provide the desired outcome, and may even have adverse effects.

Buyer Beware

I purchase my essential oils from a handful of wonderful companies that I have been dealing with for years (see Resources, page 229). Knowing your source, trusting your supplier, and training your nose (which will come with experience) are some of the best means of monitoring quality.

With the rapidly rising popularity of essential oils, deception is rampant, and unfortunately, some essential oils on the market are of poor quality. It's worth it to pay more for a reputable company's commitment to quality, because a pure and authentic product truly benefits your physical and mental health in a way that a lesser-quality product does not. I recommend calling the company whose oils you want to use and talking to someone in-the-know about the origins of their oils, production processes, and purity-testing methods.

Read the Label

The label on an essential oil bottle should list the common name of the plant (e.g., rosemary), its botanical name (*Rosmarinus officinalis*), and, if applicable, the variety or chemotype, denoted as "ct."(*Rosmarinus officinalis* ct. verbenon).

Avoid purchasing any oil marked *perfume oil, fragrance oil, scented oil,* or *essence of* — these descriptors indicate that the contents are synthetic or a synthetic blend and are of no value therapeutically.

Look for descriptors such as *ethically wildcrafted, sustainably grown,* or *certified organic.* But keep in mind that only *certified organic* has a legal definition: To be certified organic, the grower has been certified as being in compliance with strict government standards for organic production.

Certified organic essential oils are extracted from material grown without the use of pesticides, chemical fertilizers, herbicides, GMOs, or synthetic chemicals and have not been subject to irradiation and chemical sterilization. Though a certified organic essential oil is preferred, many essential oils are derived from plants that were not cultivated but responsibly wild-harvested. In other cases, the plants may have been grown under rigorous sustainability standards but not certified organic, since organic certification is often an expensive and a time-consuming process and many smaller growers just can't afford it.

The descriptors *therapeutic grade* or *aromatherapeutic grade* currently have no legal standing, but a company may use them on a product label to indicate that their essential oil is of superior quality and appropriate for therapeutic use.

Pure, therapeutic-grade essential oils can vary slightly in their scent, viscosity, and color from batch to batch. This is a sign of true quality and should be considered completely normal and natural.

What Is a Chemotype (ct.)?

Chemotypes are a phenomenon of nature whereby plants of the same species can have different chemical constituent profiles. That is, chemotypes have the same appearance as other plants of their species but different proportions of chemical components. That chemical variation may result from genetic or epigenetic factors arising from, for example, variations in light wavelengths, soil type, climate, and altitude. Because the plant has a different chemical profile, its essential oil does too.

The chemotype name — indicated with "ct." after the Latin name — identifies the predominant chemical component in the essential oil that distinguishes it from another essential oil from the same plant species. For example, rosemary essential oil in which cineole is more predominant than it is in other varieties of rosemary might be labeled "*Rosmarinus officinalis* ct. cineole." Different chemotypes will have different therapeutic properties for aromatherapy practice.

When in Doubt, Check It Out

Essential oils are highly volatile and evaporate quickly. To see this for yourself, place a drop on a sheet of plain light-colored paper, spread it around, and leave it for at least 5 hours and up to 24. A pure essential oil will evaporate, leaving either no stain or only a very light one. In contrast, a base or fatty oil, such as olive or almond, will leave a greasy stain much like potato chips kept in a paper bag. If your drop of essential oil leaves an obviously greasy stain, it has probably been diluted with a base or carrier oil, which should be indicated on the label.

Fatty oils feel greasy; essential oils do not. Rub a little olive or vegetable oil between your fingers and notice how slippery it is. An essential oil may initially seem a bit greasy, but it feels more like water and is absorbed quickly. If the essential oil feels like fatty oil, it has probably been diluted.

Essential Oils and Holistic Healing

Essential oils by themselves can only be expected to do so much. For optimal results, they should be part of a healthy lifestyle that includes a wholesome diet, ample exercise and rest, a positive attitude, good relationships, fulfilling work, fresh air and sunshine, and good stress management. This combination will almost always have a favorable influence on your health, inducing varying degrees of healing depending on the condition. Essential oils can certainly help the body and psyche heal, but there is no guarantee that they will always cure every condition for which they are indicated. No form of medicine — herbal, aromatherapeutic, allopathic, homeopathic, or otherwise — can make such a claim.

Please note that peppermint and eucalyptus essential oils should not be used by those partaking of homeopathic therapy. These oils are not to be stored near homeopathic remedies, used in conjunction with them, or diffused into the environment when ingesting the remedy, as these particular essential oils have the potential to act as antidotes.

Essential Oil Safety Tips

Essential oils are incredibly potent. They are far more concentrated than the equivalent natural flavoring in any foods or beverages you might purchase for consumption. Always treat them with the utmost respect, and don't waste them or use them haphazardly.

As long as you are careful, however, you need never worry about using essential oils. They have powerful nurturing and healing energies, and if you honor their powers, their therapeutic gifts will give you great pleasure and help you deal with many of the physical and mental challenges that might cross your life's path. There are far more advantages than disadvantages to using essential oils.

In this book, cautions for use and circumstances in which an oil should be avoided completely are indicated in the profile for each essential oil. Please read this information before using a particular oil, especially if you have concerns such as sensitive skin, if you are facing a particular medical condition or surgical situation, or if you are using them with children, with elders, or during pregnancy or lactation.

Also keep in mind that any living organism will react according to its unique genetics and current state of health, as well as environmental factors. Some people have strong reactions to particular essential oils, while others have no reaction at all, and those sensitivities can vary over time. Just because a substance is of natural origin doesn't guarantee that it's safe. Imagine the consequences of receiving a full-body massage with "all-natural" poison oak–infused oil — it's not a pretty picture!

Most folks will have a bad reaction to some plant or another at some time during their life. For the sake of safety and comfort, my advice is to observe the following tips and always err on the side of caution.

+ Use only 100 percent pure essential oils. Avoid synthetic oils and fragrance oils.

+ Wash your hands thoroughly after using undiluted essential oils.

+ Avoid contact with your eyes and mucous membranes after handling essential oils.

+ Use essential oils in a well-ventilated area.

+ Label all homemade products with the date, ingredients, and instructions for use.

+ Keep all essential oils and products made from them out of the reach of children and pets.

+ Essential oils are flammable, so use and store them away from extreme heat and open flame. If you're using the oils in a vessel designed for vaporization with a candle, follow the manufacturer's directions.

+ Avoid using essential oils of known phototoxicity prior to exposure to UV light (sunlight/tanning beds). These include lemon and bergamot. You'll sometimes also find cautions about phototoxicity with grapefruit and sweet orange essential oils, but they present a very low risk.

+ Use only essential oils externally unless otherwise indicated. Always follow the recipe directions carefully.

+ Use lower concentrations of essential oils with children, pregnant and lactating women, individuals over 70 with fragile skin, and with anyone experiencing health problems. I recommend a 0.5 to 1 percent dilution — that's 3 to 6 drops of essential oil per 1 ounce (30 ml) of carrier, be it oil, shea butter, water, or whatever.

+ Check with your medical provider or a professional aromatherapist if you have concerns.

Finally, as a general rule, do not use essential oils undiluted, as they can cause burning, skin irritation, and in some cases photosensitivity. There are a few exceptions to this rule, of course. Of the oils discussed in this book, lavender, tea tree, German and Roman chamomile, frankincense, geranium, and helichrysum may be used undiluted as spot treatments on burns, insect bites, pimples, and other skin eruptions such as small blisters, boils, or infections, as long as you don't have extremely reactive skin or have a sensitivity or allergy to the oil.

If you find that an essential oil product causes irritation of the skin, immediately wash the area and discontinue use of that oil.

Essential Oils and Pets

The formulas in this book are meant for human use only. While essential oils can be used safely with many animals, please be aware that cats and birds, in particular, are extremely sensitive to them, including to the vapors from a diffuser, and could have severe adverse reactions. When diffusing essential oils, it's highly recommended to shut cats and birds, as well as kittens and puppies under one year of age, out of the room. Never use a diffuser in a room with caged animals of any kind. When diffusing with adult dogs in the room, please provide plenty of ventilation, diffuse for only 20 to 30 minutes at a time, and make sure that they can leave the room if they wish.

Special Precautions for Children and Infants

Age-appropriate dilutions of essential oils are indicated for babies and children due to their weight and physical immaturity. The following general safety guidelines err on the side of caution, but *always* follow the specific instructions in any recipe (the quantities of essential oils may vary a bit from what I suggest here, depending on the type of recipe and percentage of body area where it will be applied). Check with a knowledgeable health-care provider or professional aromatherapist if you have concerns.

FOR NEWBORNS, BABIES, and toddlers, I recommend *only* lavender, Roman chamomile, sweet marjoram, and frankincense essential oils and use them at a rate of 6 to 8 drops per ½ cup of base (oil, cream, or lotion). Cardamom essential oil may be used as a topical indigestion remedy (see Tummy Troubles Oil, page 120), but do not apply it on or near the face as it may be too stimulating to the central nervous system and may cause breathing difficulties.

FOR CHILDREN AGED 2 TO 5 YEARS, you may use all of the oils in this book (with the exceptions noted in the caution on the facing page), but dilute them at a rate of 12 drops of essential oil per ½ cup of carrier if applying over the entire body (as in a massage oil), or up to 24 drops per ½ cup if you're using them for a more localized treatment.

FOR CHILDREN AGED 6 TO 11, use 24 drops per ½ cup of carrier if applying over the entire body (as in a massage oil), or up to 48 drops per ½ cup if you're using them for more localized treatments.

Liver Precautions

Your liver helps clear essential oils from the body. If you suffer from a liver condition, drink a lot of alcohol, have had cirrhosis of the liver or hepatitis, regularly take several medications together, take specific medications that directly affect the liver, have undergone chemotherapy, or been exposed to environmental toxins, go easy on or avoid the use of essential oils altogether. If you do use the oils, cut the suggested quantities by half and use only the gentlest ones, such as lavender, Roman chamomile, sweet orange, and frankincense.

Caution: For infants and children under age 10, do not use *Eucalyptus globulus*, *E. radiata*, *E. smithii*, or any variety of rosemary essential oil other than *Rosmarinus officinalis* ct. verbenon on or near the face, as they are too stimulating to the central nervous system and may cause breathing difficulties. Additionally, be careful using peppermint oil on or near the face of very young children; it can be a mucous membrane irritant, although the risk is low.

Emergency Response

Should you rub or splash an essential oil into your nose or eyes — which can cause excruciating pain — immediately flush the affected area with an unscented fatty oil such as olive, corn, soybean, sunflower, canola, or generic vegetable. Full-fat cream or half-and-half makes an acceptable substitute in an emergency. Using plain water does not help; essential oils are attracted to fats, not water. Should the pain continue or should severe headache or respiratory irritation develop, seek medical attention, and take the essential oil bottle with you so the medical staff knows what they are dealing with.

Some essential oils smell like candy, so keep them away from children. If more than a few drops are swallowed, severe mouth irritation, intestinal distress, or worse could result. Immediately have the person drink something fatty like half-and-half, and call a poison control center for further instructions.

Storing Essential Oils

Proper storage of essential oils is paramount to retaining freshness and potency. Air, heat, and light degrade essential oils, so store them in a cool, dark place in tightly capped, dark-colored bottles. Amber, cobalt, or dark green glass works best.

When properly stored, essential oils have a shelf life of several years. The exceptions are citrus, fir, and pine oils, which remain potent for only a year or so. Their shelf life may be extended to up to 2 years if they are refrigerated and if the bottles aren't opened too often. The longest-lasting oils, which actually improve with age, are resinous oils, such as frankincense and myrrh, and thicker oils, such as patchouli and sandalwood.

3

Aromatherapy: A Fragrant Pharmacy

Though they are the foundation of aromatherapy practice, don't let the prefix *aroma-* lead you astray. Essential oils are definitely more than mere fragrances. These botanical jewels contain serious plant medicine and offer potent healing potential. Aromatherapy is the art and science of using high-quality, therapeutic essential oils to elevate and sustain the health of your mind, body, and spirit. The oils can be administered by a number of methods, including but not limited to inhalation, massage, compresses, baths, localized topical application, gargles, liniments, salves/balms, sprays, cosmetics, and oral ingestion.

Properly prepared and applied, essential oils provide an inexpensive and pleasant way to enhance overall vitality, equilibrium, well-being, and energy, plus they can be used to help treat many specific ailments, diseases, and discomforts. Conveniently packaged and easy to use in the comfort of your own space — essential oils offer smell-good, feel-good therapy, for sure!

Aromatherapy belongs to the realm of natural therapeutics, and it shares an impressive history with other complementary natural therapies, such as herbalism, massage, reflexology, homeopathy, energy medicine, and acupuncture. The application of essential oils in cosmetics, perfumes, and medicines, as well as for spiritual, hygienic, and ritualistic purposes, dates back as far as 2800 BCE to ancient Egypt and was widespread in the Mediterranean region. Although distillation — the primary method of extracting essential oils — is credited to the Persians in the tenth century, there is evidence of distillation long before that in other ancient cultures.

During the Middle Ages, the properties of aromatic plants, including essential oils, were employed to combat infectious diseases such as the bubonic plague or "Black Death." At the time, aromatics were the best antiseptics available. By the fifteenth century, steam distillation of aromatic plants was widespread throughout Europe and by the turn of the eighteenth century, distilled essential oils were being comprehensively used in medicine, both herbal and allopathic, as were hydrosols — the watery byproducts of distillation.

The term aromatherapy was coined in 1928 by René-Maurice Gattefossé, a French chemist and perfumer whose first book, *Aromatherapie*, was published that same year. Gattefossé used the wound healing and antiseptic properties of essential oils in the care of soldiers in military hospitals during World War I.

Aromatherapy began to gain popularity in the United States in the 1980s, thanks to the tireless efforts of such notable authors, teachers, scientists, and consultants as Robert Tisserand, Kurt Schnaubelt, Michael Scholes, Marcel Lavabre, Daniel Pénoël, and others whose work propelled the wonders of essential oils and their benefits into mainstream recognition.

Our ancestors knew what we are just now rediscovering — that these scents have a powerful effect on our health, happiness, and comfort, and fortunately for us, modern scientific study of essential oils and their therapeutic properties is validating and often expanding the instinctive and trusting responses of indigenous peoples, traditional folklore, and anecdotal findings. Today's ongoing research is turning what was once viewed as an unproven "fringe modality" into a disciplined healing art that is being accepted and valued worldwide.

How Does Aromatherapy Work?

An essential oil can contain millions of molecules (some of which are quite aromatic and others not so much). These molecules easily penetrate the skin whether applied "neat" (undiluted) or diluted in a carrier, and they rapidly penetrate the mucous membranes of the respiratory system when inhaled. Through both application and inhalation, the molecules travel quickly through the capillaries and into the circulatory system, which transports them around the body.

The aromatic vapors stimulate the olfactory nerve — the only nerve in the body that is in direct contact with the external environment — and act directly on the limbic system of the brain, the area that houses memories, emotions, desires, and appetites. As the molecules travel through the body, the oils' complex array of components interact with the body's own chemistry, exerting therapeutic effects, sometimes profound ones. Their action stimulates various physiological and psychological responses, such as relief from pain, renewing of damaged skin tissue, reduction of inflammation or fever, invigoration or relaxation of the senses, release of hormones, or a positive boost in mood or cognitive ability.

The compelling benefits of pure essential oils are often nearly immediate, and you may find yourself surprised by the speed at which they work. Direct inhalation of lavender oil can quickly quell a bout of anxiety, for example, while breathing in a combination of Roman chamomile and peppermint oil can deliver blessed relief from a tension headache within minutes. A few spritzes of Sunburn Rescue Spray (page 154) deliver quick relief from a painful sunburn. All this amazing soothing plant energy conveniently packaged in a tiny bottle! That's my kind of medicine.

Interestingly, unlike with synthetic drugs or chemicals, there is evidence that essential oils do not accumulate in the human body but instead are excreted in the perspiration, breath, urine, and feces. If you constantly use the same essential oils or blends, however, it is strongly recommended that you occasionally take a break to allow your body sufficient time to properly metabolize and excrete those particular chemical constituents.

For ongoing application or inhalation, use the oil(s) or blend for 5 days, then take 2 days off. Depending on the method of administration, the particular oils used, and the genetic makeup, age, size, dietary intake, lifestyle, and overall metabolism of the individual, it can take anywhere from a few minutes to 12 hours for essential oils to be fully absorbed and 3 to 6 hours for them to be metabolized and expelled from a normal, healthy body. For an unhealthy and/or obese body, increase that to 12 to 14 hours.

Because they are highly concentrated and chemically complex, I don't generally recommend ingesting essential oils. Consumption involves direct contact with the delicate tissues of the mouth, throat, and esophagus, and the potential for extreme irritation is present. So, unless you are under the direction of a skilled aromatherapist, have undergone professional training, or are using a commercial product that contains minute amounts of essential oils specifically formulated for consumption, please do not use them internally.

In this book, essential oils are occasionally incorporated into oral preparations such as mouthwashes, gargles, toothpastes, breath sprays, or antinausea remedies. If you're using essential oils in this manner, be sure to prepare and use the recipe exactly as specified, spitting it all out, if indicated.

Dilution Guidelines

As your aromatherapy skills improve and your personal collection of essential oils expands, you may want to experiment beyond the recipes offered here. I encourage you to create your own unique formulations, so I've created a general guide to standard quantities of essential oils for various purposes.

However, you may notice that my own recipes will sometimes use more or less than the following recommendations. I do this because some conditions or situations require more or less than the standard amounts. As you become conversant with the essential oils, you will be able to gauge safe quantities for yourself, but at first it's best to be guided by the following suggestions. For more specific safety guidelines, see Essential Oil Safety Tips on page 18.

Safe and effective dilutions for most aromatherapy applications are as follows.

+   For children from 2 to 5 years old, pregnant and breastfeeding women, the elderly, and those with sensitive skin: 0.5 to 1 percent (3 to 6 drops per 2 tablespoons/1 ounce/30 ml of carrier)

+   For children over 5 years old and adults: 1 to 2 percent (6 to 12 drops per 2 tablespoons/1 ounce/30 ml of carrier)

+   For children over 12 years old and adults, in concentrated formulations designed to treat small areas of the body: 3 to 4 percent (15 to 24 drops per 2 tablespoons / 1 ounce / 30 ml of carrier)

Because pure essential oils dissolve readily in fatty solutions, the easiest and most effective way to dilute them is to combine them with a base oil or add them to a salve or balm recipe. Creams and lotions make good carriers, too. Other water-based liquids such as aloe vera juice, vinegar, vodka, witch hazel, and hydrosols can be used, but the final product must be shaken well immediately before use, as the essential oils will separate out and float to the top and thus need to be reincorporated.

Creating an Essential Oil Travel Kit

Bruises, headaches, mosquito bites, cuts and scrapes, and emotional upheavals don't just occur at home, that's for sure. It's handy to have essential oils readily available for everyday problems while you're at work, out with the kids, or on vacation. Just stock a little carrying kit with 5 ml bottles of your favorite multipurpose essential oils, along with a pair of tweezers, some cotton balls and cotton swabs, and cleansing towelettes.

I keep my kit with me all the time and use it constantly, not only for emergencies, but also for everyday enjoyment. What's in my kit? Lavender, tea tree, peppermint, clove, balsam fir, eucalyptus (*E. radiata*), rosemary (ct. verbenon), helichrysum, and sweet orange.

Suggested Dilutions for Various Methods of Application

Make adjustments according to the age and health condition of the person who will be using the product. (See pages 19 and 20 for more information.)

APPLICATION	NUMBER OF DROPS	AMOUNT OF CARRIER
Massage oil/lotion	6–12	1 ounce (30 ml) oil
Liniment	15–24	1 ounce (30 ml) vodka
Ointment (spot treatments)	24–48	2 ounces (60 ml) oil, salve, balm, lotion, cream, or gel
Compress	4–6	8 ounces (240 ml) water
Bath	5–15	1 full bath; mix the essential oils with 1 teaspoon (5 ml) salt, cream, milk, oil, honey, glycerin, or liquid soap before adding to bath
Foot/hand bath	5–10	1 gallon (3.8 L) water; mix the essential oils with 1 teaspoon (5 ml) salt, cream, milk, oil, honey, glycerin, or liquid soap before adding to water
Sitz bath	5–10	1 bath; mix the essential oils with 1 teaspoon (5 ml) oil before adding to the bath water
Facial/sinus steam	2–5	1 bowl of hot water (never boiling)
Room spray	20–30	4 ounces (120 ml) water or a 50:50 mix of water and vodka
Deodorant spray	48	8 ounces (240 ml) vodka or witch hazel
Insect repellent spray	10–12	1 ounce (30 ml) water, witch hazel, vodka, or oil
Personal inhaler sticks	12–24	Per stick
Inhalant	1–2	On a tissue or a cotton ball or pad (never use an inhalant during an asthma attack)
Gargle or mouthwash	1–2	¼ cup (60 ml) water
Diffuser/nebulizer	3–6	Always follow the manufacturer's directions
Douche	5–10	2 quarts (1.9 L) warm water

Essential Oil Measurement Conversion Chart

10 drops	¹⁄₁₀ teaspoon	¹⁄₆₀ ounce	about 0.5 ml
12.5 drops	¹⁄₈ teaspoon	¹⁄₄₈ ounce	about 0.625 ml
25 drops	¹⁄₄ teaspoon	¹⁄₂₄ ounce	about 1.25 ml
50 drops	¹⁄₂ teaspoon	¹⁄₁₂ ounce	about 2.5 ml
100 drops	1 teaspoon	¹⁄₆ ounce	about 5 ml
150 drops	1¹⁄₂ teaspoons	¹⁄₄ ounce	about 7.5 ml
300 drops	3 teaspoons	¹⁄₂ ounce	about 15 ml
600 drops	6 teaspoons	1 ounce	about 30 ml
24 teaspoons	8 tablespoons	4 ounces	about 120 ml
48 teaspoons	16 tablespoons	8 ounces	about 240 ml
96 teaspoons	32 tablespoons	16 ounces	about 470 ml

A Few More Metric Conversions

US	METRIC (APPROXIMATE)
¹⁄₄ cup	60 milliliters
¹⁄₂ cup	120 milliliters
1 cup	240 milliliters
1¹⁄₄ cups	300 milliliters
1¹⁄₂ cups	355 milliliters
2 cups	480 milliliters
2¹⁄₂ cups	600 milliliters
3 cups	710 milliliters
4 cups (1 quart)	0.95 liter

4

Essential Oil Profiles & Recipes

I have chosen a core group of essential oils, 11 of which I consider to be the most versatile and useful for treating common health concerns and supporting overall wellness, followed by 14 that are nice to have on hand but not absolutely necessary. I chose these 25 for their potent therapeutic properties and because they can safely and effectively deal with a wide range of physical and emotional issues. The majority of them are among the most inexpensive essential oils, the exceptions being frankincense CO_2, myrrh, helichrysum, and the chamomiles (Roman and German).

Following the profile of each essential oil, you'll find several recipes in which that particular oil dominates or offers noteworthy beneficial properties to the formulation. My hope is that you'll use this extraordinarily fragrant pharmacy full of delights and remedies in all aspects of your life. Today we are fortunate to be able to draw from a "global village" of aromatic healing plant essences. In addition to offering so much joy, they are capable of solving so many problems, and that, my friend, is truly something to rejoice in!

. . . and their fruit will be for food
and their leaves for healing.
EZEKIEL 47:12

THE **Top 11 Essentials**

German Chamomile

PAGE 34

Roman Chamomile

PAGE 40

Chamomile

(Matricaria recutita, syn. M. chamomilla)

The ancient Greeks called this pretty, delicate herb *kamai melon* ("ground apple") because of the apple-like scent of the daisy-like flowers and feathery leaves. Utilized primarily as a calming, tasty tea and soothing skin wash, German chamomile has a long-standing medicinal and cosmetic tradition, especially in Europe. As an herb, it is still used in many regions of the world to ease a variety of physical discomforts, especially inflammatory conditions. It's an effective aid for relieving emotional tension, sleeplessness, tension headache, and indigestion.

German chamomile essential oil is a strong anti-inflammatory that soothes any condition exhibiting heat, including gout; strained muscles, tendons, or ligaments; and irritated, inflamed skin. Possessing remarkable antiallergenic properties, it is beneficial for those suffering from hives, dermatitis, poison plant rashes, eczema, and other skin reactions.

It is an effective treatment for menstrual cramps and PMS symptoms; in fact, its genus name, *Matricaria*, refers to its role as a gynecological herb. I primarily use it in preparations to treat muscle and joint inflammation, bruises, rashes, bug bites and stings, rosacea, acne, and other skin conditions in need of powerful healing action with a cooling, calming hand.

PSYCHOLOGICAL BENEFITS: Though German chamomile essential oil is calming and soothing in cases of anxiety, insomnia, mental strain, nervous tension, and other stress-related conditions, I prefer to use Roman chamomile essential oil (page 40) for psychological or emotional concerns due to its even gentler nature, softer apple-like/floral scent, and potent relaxing, nervine, and antianxiety properties.

SAFETY DATA: Nontoxic and generally nonirritating, but it may cause dermatitis in some individuals. Avoid in cases of extremely low blood pressure.

German chamomile essential oil contains high levels of chamazulene and bisabolol, chemical components known for calming inflammation and soothing skin irritation. Chamazulene (*azul* means "blue" in Spanish), which is only produced during the process of distillation, gives the oil its unusual deep blue color.

FROM HERB TO OIL

This self-seeding annual herb, growing up to 24 inches tall and native to Europe and northern and western Asia, is now cultivated extensively around the world. The oil, produced by steam distillation of the flower heads, is a semiviscous, inky blue liquid with a pungent, sweetish-warm, almost tobacco-like aroma. The intensity of both the color and the odor can easily dominate a formula, so keep that in mind when working with this essential oil.

ESSENTIAL PROPERTIES

Cooling, anti-inflammatory, and analgesic; effective antibacterial, antifungal, and antihistamine; calming, comforting, and relieving for irritated, red, itchy skin conditions

Cooling Comfrey Balm

This is a gorgeously rich balm with the unusual spicy-sweet aroma of German chamomile and the cooling pop of peppermint. It counteracts the itch, redness, inflammation, and heat of most generic rashes and is the ultimate soother for relieving pesky insect bites and stings. It calms and comforts irritated skin tissue and encourages healing. *Safe for folks 6 years of age and older. For children aged 2 to 5, reduce the essential oils by half.*

ESSENTIAL OILS

10 ◆ German chamomile

10 ◆ peppermint

4 ◆ lavender

BASE

7 tablespoons comfrey-infused oil (page 212)

1–2 tablespoons beeswax (depending on how firm a balm you want)

4-ounce dark glass or plastic jar

TO MAKE THE BALM: Combine the comfrey oil with the beeswax in a small saucepan over low heat, or in a double boiler, and warm until the beeswax is just melted. Remove from the heat and allow to cool for 5 minutes, stirring a few times. Add the chamomile, peppermint, and lavender essential oils and stir again to thoroughly blend. Slowly pour the liquid balm into the jar. Cap, label, and set aside for 30 minutes to thicken.

Store at room temperature, away from heat and light; use within 1 year.

TO USE: Wash the affected area with mild soap and water (or try Herbal Contact Dermatitis Relief Spray, page 139). To ease intense itching, you can then apply apple cider vinegar diluted by half with purified water, if you wish. Pat dry. Massage a small amount of balm onto the rash and surrounding area. Continue twice daily until the rash is healed.

Bonus use: This formula makes an incredibly beneficial treatment for *dry* eczema and psoriasis that is accompanied by itching, peeling, flaking skin.

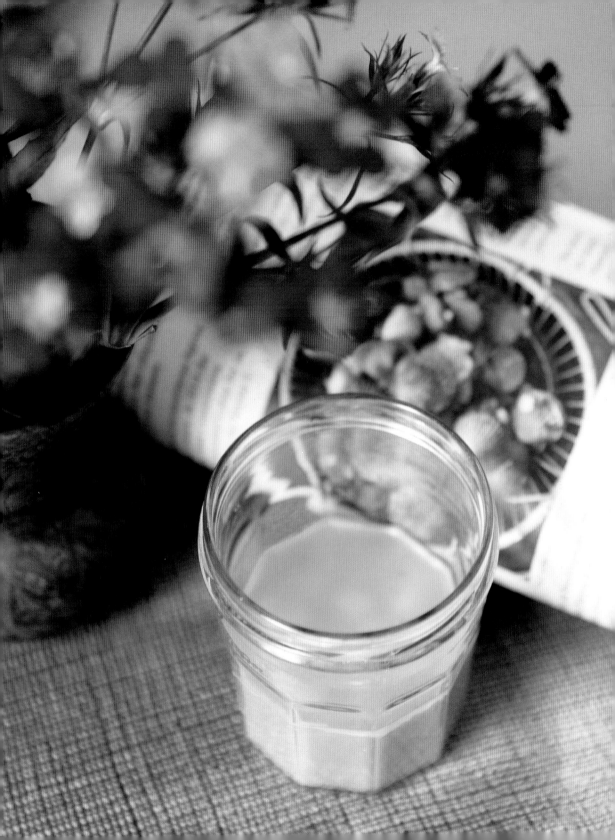

Bruise-Be-Gone Oil

An extremely powerful anti-inflammatory with a unique earthy-green-creamy aroma, this dark-hued oil gets right to the business of healing ugly bruises — pain, inflammation, tissue damage, and all. It's recommended for new bruises that are just beginning to become discolored, swollen, and hot and also for continued use on skin and muscles suffering from severe trauma. *Safe for folks 12 years of age and older. For children aged 6 to 11, reduce the essential oils by half.*

ESSENTIAL OILS

4 ⬧ German chamomile

4 ⬧ lavender

2 ⬧ lemon

2 ⬧ peppermint

BASE

1 tablespoon tamanu oil

1 tablespoon rosehip seed oil

1-ounce dark glass bottle with a dropper top

TO MAKE THE OIL: Combine the chamomile, lavender, lemon, and peppermint essential oils in the bottle, then add the tamanu and rosehip seed oils. Screw the top on the bottle and shake vigorously for 2 minutes to blend. Label the bottle and set it in a cool, dark location for 24 hours so that the oils can synergize.

Store at room temperature, away from heat and light; use within 1 year.

TO USE: Shake well before each use. Gently massage a few drops into any newly bruised area. Follow with an ice-cold compress or ice pack for 10 to 15 minutes. Do this three or four times per day for the first 2 days, until the swelling subsides. You can continue to apply this oil two or three times per day until the bruise heals. Continued application is especially recommended if the trauma was severe, with possible injury to underlying muscle tissue.

Bonus use: Use this blend to calm and comfort all manner of inflammations — skin, muscular, and joint.

Bug Bite Roll-On Remedy

This convenient, pocket-size remedy is oh-so-gentle on the skin but provides powerful anti-inflammatory, antiseptic, and analgesic properties guaranteed to take the misery out of bug bites. It promotes rapid healing of irritated, inflamed skin, too! If you don't have plantain-infused oil, you could omit it and use 2 teaspoons of calendula-infused oil instead. *Safe for folks 6 years of age and older. For infants and children up to age 5, omit all the essential oils and use only the plantain- and calendula-infused oils plus one drop of lavender.*

ESSENTIAL OILS

1 ◖ German chamomile

1 ◖ lavender

1 ◖ peppermint

1 ◖ tea tree

BASE

1 teaspoon calendula-infused oil (page 211)

1 teaspoon plantain-infused oil (page 212)

10 ml roller-ball applicator bottle

TO MAKE THE REMEDY: Combine the chamomile, lavender, peppermint, and tea tree essential oils in the bottle, then add the calendula- and plantain-infused oils. Cap and shake vigorously for 2 minutes. Label the bottle and set it in a cool, dark location for 24 hours so that the oils can synergize.

Store at room temperature, away from heat and light; use within 1 year.

TO USE: Shake well before each use. Roll a small amount onto each bug bite. Gently tap or massage into the skin. Repeat several times throughout the day, as needed for relief.

The Top 11 Essentials

MAKES 10 ML

ROMAN

Chamomile

(Chamaemelum nobile, syn. *Anthemis nobilis)*

Roman chamomile has had a medicinal reputation in Europe and especially the Mediterranean region for over 2,000 years, and it is still in widespread use. A relative of German chamomile, with the same apple-like aroma, Roman chamomile shares many of the German variety's properties and applications, even though the two herbs have a different chemistry. Due to its bitter taste, Roman chamomile is less popular as a tea, but it is a more potent digestive aid with lesser anti-inflammatory effects.

Owing to its gentleness, Roman chamomile essential oil, when used as directed, is a safe and soothing oil even for infants and young children. I often use it alone or in combination with lavender, cardamom, or frankincense essential oil in formulas designed for massage and bathing to calm irritability and induce sound sleep, as well as in topical blends designed to ease painful symptoms of teething, earache, and colic.

Because of its cooling, deeply relaxing nature, Roman chamomile is a good choice for addressing hot flashes, stress-induced skin conditions such as eczema or hives, and tension/migraine headaches. Bouts of sciatica, neuralgia, lower back pain, spasmodic muscle cramps, and menstrual cramps respond favorably as well.

PSYCHOLOGICAL BENEFITS: Roman chamomile eases anger, anxiety, fear, irritability, mental strain, nervous tension, and other stress-related conditions. It's wonderfully beneficial during the emotional swings of PMS and menopause.

SAFETY DATA: Nontoxic and generally nonirritating, but it may cause dermatitis in some individuals.

EO Extra: Roman Chamomile

Combine 2 drops of Roman chamomile and 4 drops lavender essential oil with ¼ cup of aloe vera juice in a spritzer bottle. This mist will comfort and speed healing to skin damaged by sunburn, windburn, or simple dehydration, and even work wonderfully well as a skin toner to help calm and heal rosacea and acne pimples. May be used on very young children.

FROM HERB TO OIL

A perennial herb with a multibranched hairy stem, Roman chamomile has flowers a bit larger than those of German chamomile. It is native to southern and western Europe and has naturalized in North America. The essential oil is produced by steam distillation of the flower heads. Its intensely sweet, fruity-floral, warm, apple-like herbaceous scent can easily dominate a formula.

ESSENTIAL PROPERTIES

Known as the "flower of tranquility"; gentle, cooling pain reliever; exceptional digestive and calming agent; remarkable antispasmodic, with relaxant and sedative properties; specific for infants, the elderly, and those with sensitive skin in need of healing with a soft touch.

Pure and Gentle Herbal Baby Oil

With skin-soothing, calming herbal extracts and a subtle apple-floral scent, this blend provides a conditioning, protective barrier that seals in valuable moisture while serving as an effective healing aid for minor irritations of a baby's delicate skin. Use as a full-body massage oil, bath oil, foot rub, or diaper rash preventive oil.

ESSENTIAL OILS

2 ◆ lavender

2 ◆ Roman chamomile

BASE

¼ cup calendula-infused oil (page 211) or jojoba oil

2-ounce plastic squeeze bottle or dark glass bottle with a pump or dropper top

TO MAKE THE OIL: Combine the lavender and chamomile essential oils in the bottle, then add the calendula oil. Screw the top on the bottle and shake vigorously for 2 minutes to blend. Label the bottle and set it in a cool, dark location for 24 hours so that the oils can synergize.

Store at room temperature, away from heat and light; use within 1 year (or 2 years if you used jojoba oil).

TO USE: Shake well before each use. Massage a small amount into baby's skin, as desired. For use as a bath oil, add ½ to 1 teaspoon to a small tub full of warm water and swish to blend with your hands before placing your child in the tub. After bathing, pat baby's skin dry, and follow with an application of this same oil or your favorite natural baby lotion.

Bonus uses: For those of you with ultra-sensitive skin, no matter what your age, this gentle oil will be your skin's best friend. It also can serve as a healing aid for new bruises, insect bites and stings, sunburn, windburn, or dry, cracked, or chapped skin.

Cool-the-Flash Mist

That powerful surge of heat that spreads throughout your body, seemingly emanating from your core, can wreak havoc with your sleep patterns, emotions, and confidence about being in public places. If you're a woman over 40, you've probably experienced at least a few (if not many more) of these often inopportunely timed episodes.

This recipe contains cooling, aromatic essential oils traditionally used to subdue surging surface heat and skin inflammation, and aid in balancing hormonal mood swings, nervous tension, and exhaustion. Just mist it on, deeply breathe in the soothing vapors, and feel better fast! Keep a bottle handy wherever you go.

ESSENTIAL OILS

8 ◆ Roman chamomile

6 ◆ lavender

6 ◆ lemon

4 ◆ geranium

2 ◆ peppermint

BASE

¾ cup purified water

¼ cup unflavored vodka

½ teaspoon vegetable glycerin

8-ounce plastic or dark glass spritzer bottle

TO MAKE THE MIST: Combine the water, vodka, and glycerin in the bottle, then add the chamomile, lavender, lemon, geranium, and peppermint essential oils. Screw the top on the bottle and shake vigorously to blend. Label the bottle and allow the spray to synergize for at least 1 hour.

Store at room temperature, away from heat and light; use within 1 year.

TO USE: Shake well before use. When in need of a hot flash chill-down, lightly mist your face and exposed skin and breathe deeply. Use as desired. The spray feels ultra-cool if refrigerated!

Bonus uses: This blend can serve as a light floral-citrusy room freshener to eliminate stale odors, as well as a pillow mist to help you relax before you nod off to sleep.

The Top 11 Essentials

MAKES 8 OUNCES (240 ML)

Chamomile Comfort Teething Oil

Teething usually begins around 4 to 7 months of age when the first "milk teeth" arrive. Some infants teethe without discomfort, but for others teething can be painful and distressing. Common symptoms include inflammation and soreness of the gums, increased irritability, drooling, chin rash, a desire to gnaw everything, difficulty sleeping, earache, diaper rash, and low-grade fever.

This gentle remedy will help soothe irritated gums, jawbone, and facial muscles while also calming crankiness.

ESSENTIAL OILS
6 ♦ Roman chamomile or lavender

BASE
2 tablespoons almond, jojoba, or sunflower oil

1-ounce dark glass storage bottle with a dropper top

TO MAKE THE OIL: Combine the chamomile essential oil and your base oil of choice in the bottle. Screw the top on the bottle and shake vigorously to blend. Label the bottle.

Store at room temperature, away from heat and light; use within 1 year (or 2 years if you used jojoba oil).

TO USE: Shake well before each use. Ever-so-gently, massage a few drops of this formula on the baby's exterior cheeks, jawline, and just below the ear, being careful to avoid the eye area. Hold a warm, damp washcloth on the area until it is almost cool. Repeat several times per day.

Bonus use: This blend doubles as a calming, sleep-inducing massage oil. Place a few drops in the palm of your hand, rub your palms together to warm the oil, and then gently massage the oil into the child's feet and ankles. It makes you more relaxed as well!

MAKES 1 OUNCE (30 ML)

Simple Earache Remedy

Simple earaches can be effectively relieved with a gentle, antiseptic essential oil blend and a warm compress or heating pad. This recipe is just what the herb doc ordered! *Safe for folks over 6 years of age. For children aged 2 to 5, reduce the quantity of essential oils by half.*

ESSENTIAL OILS

6 ◆ Roman chamomile

4 ◆ lavender

2 ◆ tea tree

BASE

2 tablespoons almond, jojoba, extra-virgin olive, or sunflower oil

1-ounce dark glass bottle with a dropper top

Caution: Never apply essential oils, diluted or undiluted, directly into the ear!

TO MAKE THE REMEDY: Combine the chamomile, lavender, and tea tree essential oils in the bottle, then add your base oil of choice. Screw the top on the bottle and shake vigorously for 2 minutes to blend. Label the bottle and set it in a cool, dark location for 24 hours so that the oils can synergize.

Store at room temperature, away from heat and light; use within 1 year (or 2 years if you used jojoba oil).

TO USE: Shake well before using. Rub a few drops around the outside of the painful ear and down the side of the neck over the lymph nodes. Gently massage for a minute or so. Then add a few drops of the oil blend to a cotton ball and place it in the external opening of the ear. Apply a very warm, slightly damp compress or small microwave-activated "moist heat" heating pad over the ear (just make sure it isn't uncomfortably hot), and hold it in place for 10 minutes. Repeat three times per day, continuing the treatment for several days after the pain is gone.

The Top 11 Essentials

MAKES 1 OUNCE (30 ML)

Clove Bud

(Syzygium aromaticum, syn. *Eugenia caryophyllata)*

Cloves have played an important role in the spice trade since the sixteenth century. They have been employed for myriad purposes, such as to fight skin infections, ease digestive upset, cover up body odor, numb a toothache, improve bad breath, get rid of intestinal parasites, allay nausea, ease the pain of childbirth (when steeped in wine), season both savory and sweet edibles, and fragrance the home. Before the days of refrigeration, cloves were used to preserve meat and/or improve the taste of meat that was past its prime.

The stimulating heat and analgesic qualities of clove essential oil comfort while also getting sluggish circulation moving, making it quite beneficial for those suffering from chronically cold hands and feet, including vascular disorders such as Raynaud's disease. As well, it delivers welcome relief to cold, stiff, achy muscles and arthritic joints. In formulations designed to combat bacterial, viral, and fungal infections such as colds, flu, bronchitis, sinusitis, boils, acne, nail fungus, and athlete's foot, it boosts the effectiveness of the other essential oils in the blend.

PSYCHOLOGICAL BENEFITS: Clove imparts a sense of cheerfulness, optimism, joy, and courage.

SAFETY DATA: Irritating to the skin and mucous membranes; may cause dermatitis. Repeated topical application with minimal dilution, such as using the oil to ease toothache or eliminate warts, can result in extreme contact sensitization for some individuals. For inhalation, whether in a room spray or diffuser, it's best used highly diluted and blended with lighter, brighter essential oils, due to its irritating properties and hot nature. Please use as directed in recipes, or in low dilutions of 0.5 percent or less. Avoid if you are pregnant or breastfeeding. Do not ingest clove essential oil if you are using anticoagulants, following major surgery, or if you suffer from peptic ulcer, hemophilia, or another bleeding disorder.

Traditionally used to temporarily relieve toothache pain, clove essential oil has been approved by the American Dental Association as an anesthetic. Its spicy heat and antiseptic, deodorizing properties make it a wonderful additive to homemade toothpastes, powders, and gargles, but remember — a little goes a long, long way.

FROM HERB TO OIL

Cloves are the dried woody buds of a slender evergreen tree that has been cultivated worldwide for over 2,000 years. Once established, clove trees can bear their fragrant buds for at least a century. Today they are grown primarily in Madagascar, Indonesia, Sri Lanka, and Zanzibar, where the oil is steam-distilled from the immature flower buds.

Clove bud essential oil is pale yellow and has a warm, sweet-spicy, pungent, slightly woody, almost sharp odor with a peculiar fruity-fresh top note. The oil distilled from the leaves contains more of the harsh compound eugenol and is best avoided. When blending clove bud with other essential oils, keep in mind that its intense scent can quickly dominate the blend. Always use a respectful hand with this oil, not just because of the tenacious aroma, but because of its hot, potentially irritating nature. Less is indeed more with clove!

ESSENTIAL PROPERTIES

Hot and powerful circulatory stimulant; broad-spectrum antibacterial, antiviral, and antifungal; excellent pain reliever; digestive aid and breath freshener

Traditional Clove Toothache Remedy

Clove essential oil contains eugenol, a strong analgesic and antiseptic. It has been used for centuries to help alleviate pain associated with dental cavities and oral infection. *Safe for folks 12 years of age and older.*

ESSENTIAL OIL

1 ◊ clove

BASE

2 ◊ almond, sunflower, extra-virgin olive, or unrefined coconut oil

Nonreactive container, such as stainless steel teaspoon or a shot glass

TO MAKE AND USE: Combine the clove essential oil with your base oil of choice in the container. Stir with a cotton swab, then dab directly onto the aching tooth and gently massage the surrounding gum area. Expect to experience temporary numbness in the affected area. Repeat the treatment up to three times per day for up to 1 week. If the pain persists, see your dentist as soon as possible.

Caution: Clove oil is very strong and a potential skin irritant. If you experience an intolerable burning sensation or lingering irritation, stop treatment immediately and rinse out your mouth with cream, half-and-half, whole milk, or vegetable oil several times until the irritation abates.

Wart-Be-Gone Compound

This blend effectively treats both common and plantar warts. Caused by a type of human papillomavirus, common warts (*Verruca vulgaris*) are small, firm, rough, raised hard growths, occasionally having a tiny black dot at the core, that affect the outer layer of the skin, or epidermis. They are usually found on the backs of hands and fingers but may occur anywhere on the skin. Plantar warts (*Verruca plantaris*) develop on the soles of the feet but become flattened and embedded due to pressure caused by walking on them, and they often become quite painful.

I use apple cider vinegar as the base of this formula because it contains malic acid, an exfoliating chemical that dissolves the top dead layer of epidermal cells and softens tough tissue, allowing the antiviral essential oils to penetrate more easily and do their job more effectively. *Safe for folks 6 years of age and older. This formula is not intended for use on genital warts.*

ESSENTIAL OILS

5 ● clove

5 ● tea tree

4 ● lavender

4 ● lemon

BASE

2 tablespoons apple cider vinegar (preferably organic and unpasteurized)

1-ounce dark glass bottle with a dropper top

TO MAKE THE BLEND: Combine the clove, tea tree, lavender, and lemon essential oils in the bottle, then add the vinegar. Screw the top on the bottle and shake vigorously to blend. Label the bottle and allow the formula to synergize for at least 1 hour.

Store at room temperature, away from heat and light; use within 1 year.

TO USE: Shake well before use. Apply 1 drop to each wart and massage in well; cover with a bandage. Avoid getting on surrounding skin as much as possible. Use twice daily. Warts are stubborn creatures. Applying this blend *consistently* is key to dissolving and ultimately eradicating warts. If irritation develops, discontinue use.

The Top 11 Essentials

MAKES 1 OUNCE (30 ML)

Stephanie's Essential Heal-All Oil

With its fresh, herbaceous, medicinal aroma, this formula — one of my tried-and-true favorites — will aid in healing just about any minor to moderate skin injury, as well as relieving headaches, easing sinus pressure, and comforting stiff muscles and joints. Although hot, spicy clove essential oil seemingly plays a minor role, I include it for its remarkably potent antibacterial, antiviral, anti-fungal, and analgesic properties. *Safe for folks 12 years of age and older. Children between the ages of 6 and 11 can use this formula by the drop, as directed, but not on their face or chest for any reason due to the inclusion of eucalyptus.*

ESSENTIAL OILS

8 ◆ rosemary (ct. verbenon)

8 ◆ tea tree

4 ◆ eucalyptus (species *globulus*, *radiata*, or *smithii*)

4 ◆ peppermint

3 ◆ clove

3 ◆ lavender

BASE

¼ cup almond, extra-virgin olive, sunflower, or jojoba oil

2-ounce dark glass bottle with a dropper top

Caution: Due to the concentration of essential oils, use this oil blend only on areas in need of relief, not as a whole-body massage oil.

TO MAKE THE OIL: Combine the rosemary, tea tree, eucalyptus, peppermint, clove, and lavender essential oils in the bottle, then add your base oil of choice. Screw the top on the bottle and shake vigorously for 2 minutes to blend. Label the bottle and set it in a cool, dark location for 24 hours so that the oils can synergize.

Store at room temperature, away from heat and light; use within 1 year (or 2 years if you used jojoba oil).

TO USE: Shake well before using. For cuts and scrapes, apply a few drops of this formula to the injury twice per day to discourage infection and speed healing. Apply a bandage as desired. For sinus pain and pressure related to colds and flu, rub a few drops of this fabulous oil onto cheekbones, temples, throat, and chest to open respiratory channels and the sinuses. To ease headaches, massage a drop or two into the temples and on the nape of neck. For stiff joints and muscles, use as a spot-treatment massage oil.

MAKES 2 OUNCES (60 ML)

Eucalyptus

(Eucalyptus globulus, E. radiata, E. smithii)

Both the crushed leaves and essential oil of eucalyptus have long been used by Australian Aboriginal tribes to treat fungal conditions, burns, insect bites, wounds, infection (especially respiratory), muscular pain, congestion, and feverish tropical diseases such as malaria, cholera, and typhoid. For centuries, people burned the leaves as fumigation to relieve fever and repel disease-carrying insects.

The essential oil is one of nature's most powerful antibiotics, destroying not only a wide range of bacteria but also fungi and viruses. I tend to prefer *E. radiata*, but all three can be used to relieve and/or fend off colds, flu, and respiratory and throat infections. Eucalyptus is an amazing decongestant and mucolytic, meaning it helps thin mucus, which is why it is added to many commercial vapor rubs. It is also often used to treat herpes and chickenpox, and it is most beneficial in healing wounds and sores and eradicating athlete's foot, nail fungus, ringworm, lice, and scabies.

Eucalyptus essential oil is initially cool upon inhalation but actually warming upon the skin, making it quite effective in liniments used to ease the pain of achy or stiff muscles, stressed tendons and ligaments, sciatica, and arthritic joints. Like clove, it gets sluggish circulation moving.

PSYCHOLOGICAL BENEFITS:

Eucalyptus is generally uplifting to the psyche. It is said to open, expand, and stimulate the mind, assisting with decision making. It lends clarity and energy when you are emotionally fatigued, confused, or fearful of change.

SAFETY DATA: Generally nontoxic, nonirritating (in dilution), and nonsensitizing. Avoid use of *E. globulus* essential oil if you are pregnant or breastfeeding. (*E. radiata* and *E. smithii*, the gentlest of all eucalyptus species, are safe for pregnant and breastfeeding women and are the best choices for seniors and anyone with sensitive skin.) Do not use *E. globulus*, *E. radiata*, or *E. smithii* essential oils on or near the face for infants or children under 10, as they are too stimulating to the central nervous system and may cause breathing difficulties. Please note that eucalyptus essential oils are *not* compatible with homeopathic treatment.

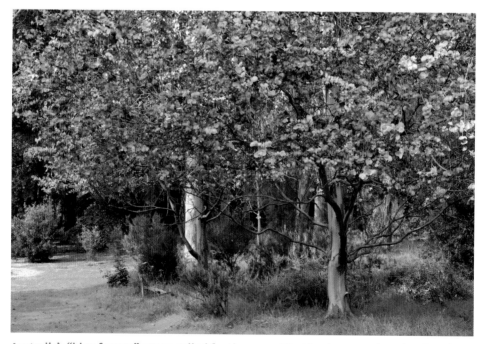

Australia's "blue forests" are so called for the smog-like blue haze produced on hot days by the essential oil vaporizing from eucalyptus leaves.

FROM HERB TO OIL

Growing to over 250 feet tall, *E. globulus*, known as blue gum eucalyptus, is an attractive evergreen with bluish-green oval leaves. *E. smithii*, or gully gum eucalyptus, is also quite tall, but with gray-green leaves. *E. radiata*, also known as narrow-leaved peppermint eucalyptus, which matures to approximately half the size of *E. globulus*, produces green to gray-green leaves.

The essential oil is produced by steam distillation of the fresh or partially dried leaves and young twigs. It is a clear to very pale yellow liquid with a fresh, pungent, somewhat harsh, and strongly camphorous aroma. *E. globulus* is the most potent of the three described in this book. *E. radiata* has a milder aroma and gentler nature upon the skin but offers a surprisingly powerful antiviral capacity. *E. smithii* has a dry, light odor and is gentle on the skin as well.

ESSENTIAL PROPERTIES

Powerfully antibacterial, antiviral, and antifungal; remarkable decongestant/expectorant; energizing, warming, and stimulating for circulation; recommended pain reliever for muscular and arthritic complaints; valuable insect repellent and parasiticide

The Top 11 Essentials

"Pure Hands" Sanitizing Spray

With a bright, uplifting, green-minty-citrus aroma, this wonderfully effective and synthetic chemical–free hand sanitizer combines several essential oils that offer antibacterial, antiviral, and antifungal properties. It's one of my must-have natural health-care products! *Safe for folks 12 years of age and older.*

ESSENTIAL OILS

8 ◆ eucalyptus (species *globulus*, *radiata*, or *smithii*)

6 ◆ peppermint

6 ◆ rosemary (ct. verbenon or nonchemotype specific)

6 ◆ tea tree

4 ◆ lemon

BASE

¼ cup unflavored vodka

¼ cup purified water

½ teaspoon vegetable glycerin

4-ounce plastic or dark glass spritzer bottle

TO MAKE THE SPRAY: Combine the vodka, water, and glycerin in the bottle, then add the eucalyptus, peppermint, rosemary, tea tree, and lemon essential oils. Screw the top on the bottle and shake vigorously to blend. Label the bottle and allow the spray to synergize for at least 1 hour.

Store at room temperature, away from heat and light; use within 1 year.

TO USE: Shake well before each use. Use after washing your hands for an extra layer of protection, or carry a small bottle with you as a hand sanitizer for times when washing is not possible. Avoid direct contact with the eyes, nose, and mouth.

Bonus uses: Use this blend as a disinfecting room spray during cold and flu season, a bathroom deodorizer, and a countertop cleanser/sanitizer for the kitchen and bathroom.

Sore Muscle Bath Salts

Soothing, relaxing salvation for sore muscles, stiffness, and achy joints — a long, warm, skin-softening soak in this salty blend is the perfect way to end your day on a comfortable note. *Safe for folks 12 years of age and older.*

ESSENTIAL OILS

- 4 ◊ eucalyptus (species *globulus*, *radiata*, or *smithii*)

- 4 ◊ lavender

- 4 ◊ rosemary (ct. verbenon or nonchemotype specific)

BASE

- 1 cup Epsom salt or sea salt

- ½ cup baking soda

TO MAKE THE BATH SALTS: Combine the Epsom salt and baking soda in a medium bowl and mix well. Add the eucalyptus, lavender, and rosemary essential oils and stir well to combine.

TO USE: Close the bathroom door so that you capture the healing vapors. Fill the tub with very warm water. Add the bath salts to the tub and swish with your hands to thoroughly disperse the essential oils. Step in and soak for 20 to 30 minutes. Pat dry, and follow with an application of your favorite natural body lotion or cream. Ahhh . . . don't you feel better?

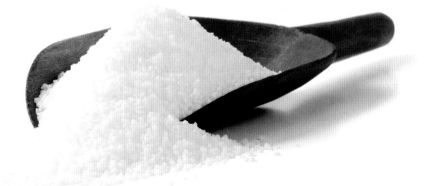

Bonus use: If you're suffering from head congestion or respiratory tightness, the vapors emanating from this bath will bring blessed relief to your ailing body.

Open Sinus!

Specifically formulated for those of you with a delicate constitution and sensitive skin, this gentle, skin-friendly blend delivers stimulating, antibacterial, antiviral, mucolytic (mucus-thinning) properties to help open clogged sinuses and relieve chest congestion in an easy-to-use roller-ball applicator. Consider it your personal bottle of respiratory therapy. *Safe for folks 12 years of age and older. To ensure the utmost gentleness, you must use the exact species and chemotypes of the essential oils specified below.*

ESSENTIAL OILS

4 ◆ eucalyptus (species *radiata* or *smithii*)

2 ◆ rosemary (ct. verbenon)

1 ◆ peppermint

1 ◆ thyme (ct. linalool)

BASE

2 teaspoons jojoba or fractionated coconut oil

10 ml roller-ball applicator bottle

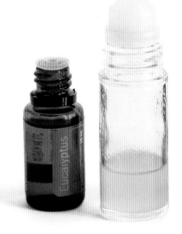

TO MAKE THE BLEND: Combine the eucalyptus, rosemary, peppermint, and thyme essential oils in the bottle, then add your base oil of choice. Cap the bottle and shake vigorously for 2 minutes. Label the bottle and set it in a cool, dark location for 24 hours so that the oils can synergize.

Store at room temperature, away from heat and light; use within 2 years.

TO USE: Shake well before each use. Roll a little oil onto your upper lip area (not directly on your lips), temples, and cheekbones. Massage in well. Next, roll some into one palm, rub your palms together to warm the oil, then close your eyes and inhale the vapors from your cupped hands (inhale through your mouth if your nose is stuffed up). Breathe slowly and deeply for a few minutes. Repeat several times throughout the day, as desired. You can also rub some of the oil into your feet, where the therapeutic properties will be absorbed via thousands of sweat glands (roll a bit into palms, then apply to your feet). Avoid direct contact with eyes, nose, and mouth.

Hot and Cold Analgesic Massage Oil

Simultaneously warming and chilling, this blend is the ultimate soother for an inflamed, aching back. It can also be used for muscle pain, fatigue, inflammation, soreness, stiffness, or tension in any part of the body. It brings wonderful relief to fresh bruises, too! Its aroma is herbaceous with a hint of spice, and not overly medicinal. *Safe for folks 12 years of age and older. Due to the essential oil concentration, this blend should not be used as a whole-body massage oil. Apply to localized areas of intense pain only.*

ESSENTIAL OILS

18 ◆ eucalyptus (species *globulus*, *radiata*, or *smithii*)

18 ◆ peppermint

14 ◆ rosemary (ct. verbenon or nonchemotype specific)

5 ◆ German chamomile

5 ◆ clove

BASE

½ cup jojoba, almond, sunflower, or extra-virgin olive oil

4-ounce plastic squeeze bottle or dark glass bottle with a pump or dropper top

TO MAKE THE OIL: Combine the eucalyptus, peppermint, rosemary, chamomile, and clove essential oils in the bottle, then add your base oil of choice. Screw the top on the bottle and shake vigorously for 2 minutes to blend. Label the bottle and set it in a cool, dark location for 24 hours so that the oils can synergize.

Store at room temperature, away from heat and light; use within 1 year (or 2 years if you used jojoba oil).

TO USE: Shake well before each use. If possible, have a friend or partner massage this soothing remedy, once or twice per day, into muscles that are sore and achy. Using it on skin that is prewarmed from a bath, shower, or heating pad encourages penetration of the oil.

Bonus uses: This oil can also ease pain and inflammation in arthritic joints, or you can use a few drops to soothe and deodorize tired, aching feet.

The Top 11 Essentials

MAKES 4 OUNCES (120 ML)

Raven's Wings Foot Gel for Colds and Flu

Did you know that your feet have approximately 250,000 sweat glands? That's a heck of a lot of entry points for therapeutic essential oils, and one of my favorite ways to apply them is with a good, relaxing foot rub. If you can enlist the aid of a friend or loved one, all the better!

When I'm suffering from a bad cold or flu — or even just feeling like I'm about to succumb — I reach for this fresh, uplifting formula. It's chock-full of antiviral, antiseptic, and respiratory-channel-clearing properties. In short, it will help your symptoms fly away on raven's wings. This highly penetrative blend fortifies resistance and general immunity and keeps microbes at bay, so you might want to use it daily prior to cold and flu season. Dang good stuff! *Safe for folks 12 years of age and older. This is an aromatherapeutically concentrated formula, so use only as directed.*

ESSENTIAL OILS
- 12 ♦ eucalyptus (species *globulus, radiata*, or *smithii*)
- 10 ♦ peppermint
- 10 ♦ rosemary (ct. verbenon or nonchemotype specific)
- 8 ♦ tea tree
- 4 ♦ balsam fir
- 2 ♦ cinnamon bark
- 2 ♦ clove

BASE
- ½ teaspoon unflavored vodka
- 4 tablespoons commercially prepared aloe vera gel
- 2-ounce dark glass or plastic jar

TO MAKE THE GEL: Combine the vodka with the eucalyptus, peppermint, rosemary, tea tree, balsam fir, cinnamon, and clove essential oils in a small glass or stainless steel bowl; a custard cup works well. Mix thoroughly, then add the aloe vera gel and stir vigorously to blend. Pour the gel into the jar, cap, and label. Allow product to synergize for 24 hours prior to use.

Store the gel in the refrigerator, where it will keep for up to 6 months.

TO USE: Gently stir before each use, as the essential oils may separate from the aloe vera gel. Spoon ½ teaspoon of gel into your hand and gently massage into the sole of each foot and between the toes. Afterward, put on socks. Do this two or three times per day. I also like to massage a small amount of gel into my chest, as I find that the scent and healing properties ease sinus and lung congestion. Avoid direct contact with the eyes, nose, and mouth.

Bonus uses: This gel also aids in healing cuts, scrapes, acne pimples, boils, insect bites, bedsores or skin ulcers, blisters, cold sores (oral), shingles, and any minor to moderate skin infections. Simply apply a small amount two or three times per day.

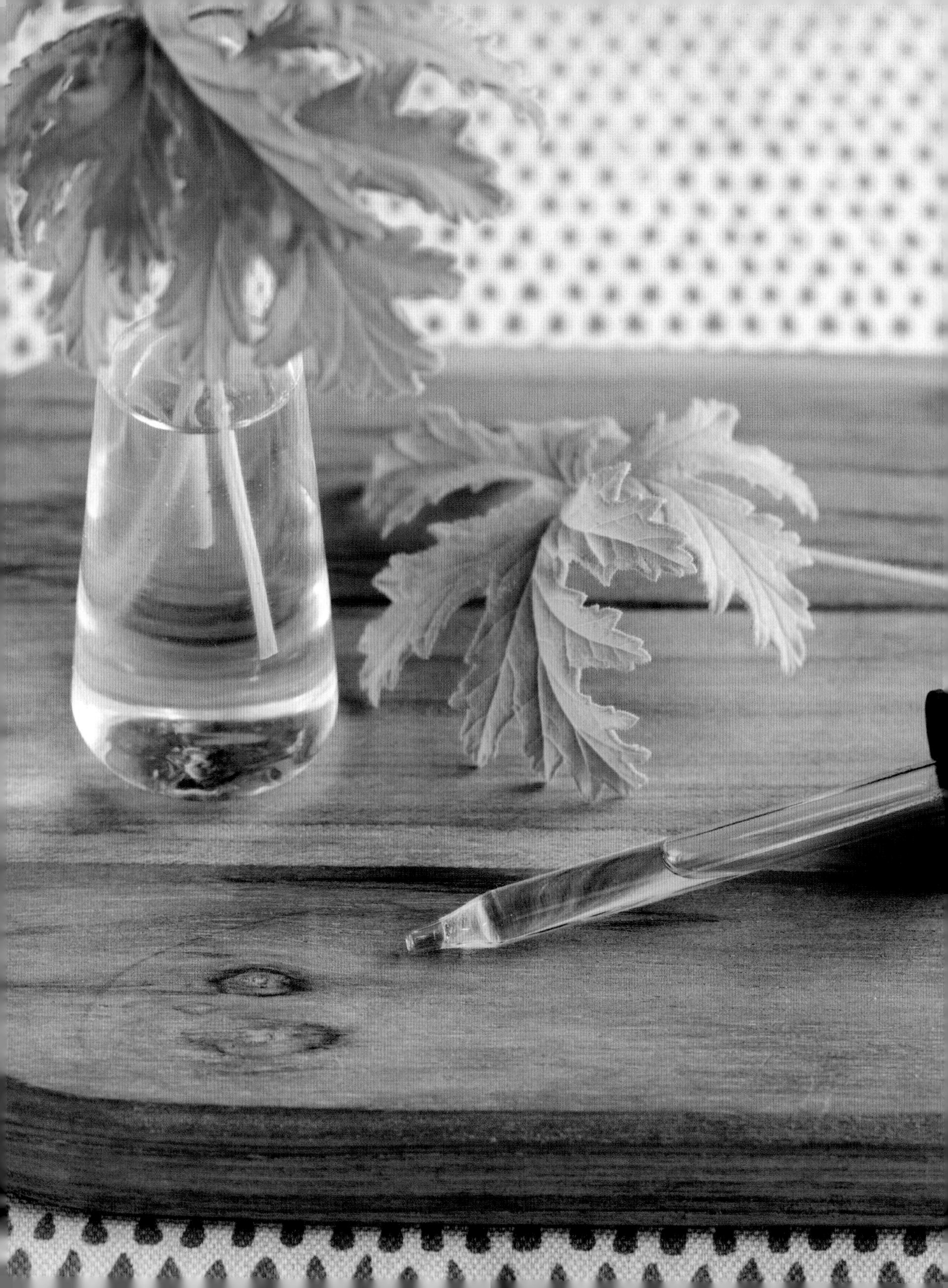

Geranium

(Pelargonium graveolens; P. × asperum)

This highly aromatic plant has long been adored for the delicious complexity of its bouquet; seventeenth-century Europeans loved it so much that they developed hundreds of hybrids. Geranium leaves make a soothing rose-flavored tea and are prized for their use in making a fragrant body wash, natural deodorant, and effective insect repellent. They can also be used to promote healing for a broad range of conditions, from dysentery and cholera to hemorrhoids and infections of the skin.

As a soothing astringent, geranium essential oil tones and tightens the skin and astringes excess moisture, making it an excellent choice for weeping eczema, psoriasis, edema, and hemorrhoids. Considered a "beautifying oil," it benefits the health of both the skin and scalp by balancing sebum (oil) production in all skin types. With its parasiticidal properties, it is also helpful in blends formulated to combat nail fungus, athlete's foot, ringworm, and lice.

For those with impaired circulation or vascular disorders, such as Raynaud's disease, couperose skin (skin exhibiting diffuse redness due to dilated capillaries), or varicose and spider veins, geranium will help regulate blood flow.

PSYCHOLOGICAL BENEFITS: "Balancing" is the best way to describe this oil. It seems to bestow upon you what you need. It is gently refreshing, uplifting, calming, grounding, and centering, yet not sedating. The aroma encourages feelings of peace and harmony, while uncluttering a chaotic mind. It is useful for treating depression, nervous tension, anxiety, and restlessness, and it's a wonderful choice for those moving through a stressful menopause.

SAFETY DATA: Generally considered nontoxic, nonirritating, and nonsensitizing, but it may cause contact dermatitis in hypersensitive individuals.

Sometimes called "the woman's oil," geranium essential oil is indeed a special gift for women because of its positive regulatory actions upon the hormones secreted by the adrenal cortex. This makes it a valuable remedy for problems caused by fluctuating hormone levels, including PMS, engorged and/or painful breasts, and menopausal symptoms such as hot flashes and vaginal dryness.

FROM HERB TO OIL

A native of South Africa, this tender perennial fuzzy shrub has pointed leaves and clusters of small pink, red, or white flowers. The entire plant is aromatic. The genus name *Pelargonium* derives from the Greek *pelargos*, "stork," in reference to the herb's long, bill-like seeds. Over 250 varieties of scented geraniums are cultivated all over the world. *P. graveolens* is the name most often found on commercial essential oil labels, though it is unlikely to be the true botanical source.

The leaves, green stems, and flowers are harvested at the start of the flowering period and steam-distilled to produce the clear, greenish essential oil. It has a rather heady, tenacious (even cloying) earthy-green rose-like scent.

When purchasing geranium essential oil, you may have a choice between Egyptian, Chinese, and Bourbon varieties. The Egyptian, which tends to be the least expensive, has a less-sweet, grassy-rose aroma. The Chinese smells like typical geranium, being rosy-earthy-green. The Bourbon is the cream of the crop, with an exquisitely clean and sweet scent, but it is also the most expensive. They all work equally well in my recipes; it's just a matter of taste and budget.

ESSENTIAL PROPERTIES

Gentle astringent and diuretic, good for water retention/edema; antibacterial and antifungal; mild anti-inflammatory and moderate circulatory stimulant; promotes wound healing; cooling; emotionally and physically balancing; valuable insect repellent and parasiticide

Geranium Oil or Rose Oil?

Geranium essential oil is sometimes confused with rose (*Rosa damascena*) essential oil, due to its rose-like scent and the fact that it's occasionally labeled "rose geranium." In fact, geranium oil is frequently used to adulterate and extend real rose oil, and it is the starting point in the manufacture of synthetic rose oil.

Skeeter Guard Insect Repellent Spray

Although formulated with a low concentration of essential oils, this tough-on-bugs, skin-friendly repellent has a fragrance that appeals to us but offends pesky insects. It's wonderfully effective at keeping hungry bugs at bay. (The mildly to moderately hungry ones, at least — from my experience, no all-natural repellent has yet been invented that will stop truly voracious mosquitos!) *Safe for use by folks 12 years of age and older.*

ESSENTIAL OILS

14 ◆ geranium

12 ◆ eucalyptus (species *globulus*, *radiata*, or *smithii*)

10 ◆ lavender

8 ◆ rosemary (ct. verbenon or nonchemotype specific)

4 ◆ peppermint

BASE

½ teaspoon vegetable glycerin

1 cup commercially prepared witch hazel

8-ounce plastic or dark glass spritzer bottle

TO MAKE THE SPRAY: Combine the geranium, eucalyptus, lavender, rosemary, and peppermint essential oils in the bottle, then add the glycerin and witch hazel. Screw the top on the bottle and shake vigorously to blend. Label the bottle and allow the spray to synergize for at least 1 hour.

Store at room temperature, away from heat and light; use within 1 year.

TO USE: Shake well before each use. Apply liberally to skin as needed. You may need to reapply it every 20 to 30 minutes. May be sprayed on clothing.

Bonus use: This spray doubles as a refreshing, uplifting, aromatic room mist.

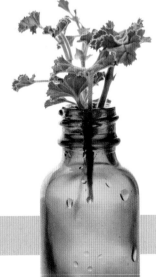

MAKES 8 OUNCES (240 ML)

Happy Feet and Hands Antifungal Drops

This herbal oil blend, with its unusual yet pleasing medicinal aroma, works double duty, eliminating the scourge of both athlete's foot and nail fungus. It also calms and soothes redness and itching, helps heal infection, conditions cracked or peeling skin, and fights odor. *Safe for folks 12 years of age and older. This is an aromatherapeutically concentrated formula, so use only by the drop as directed.*

ESSENTIAL OILS

15 ◊ geranium

10 ◊ lavender

10 ◊ tea tree

5 ◊ lemon

5 ◊ thyme (ct. linalool or nonchemotype specific)

3 ◊ German chamomile

BASE

¼ cup jojoba, almond, extra-virgin olive, or sunflower oil

2-ounce dark glass bottle with a dropper top

Bonus uses: This formula is also effective as an aid in healing cuts and scrapes as it helps prevent infection, speeds skin tissue repair, and minimizes scar formation. Apply by the drop. It delivers blessed comfort for painful bruises, too.

TO MAKE THE DROPS: Combine the geranium, lavender, tea tree, lemon, thyme, and chamomile essential oils in the bottle, then add your base oil of choice. Screw the top on the bottle and shake vigorously for 2 minutes to blend. Label the bottle and set it in a cool, dark location for 24 hours so that the oils can synergize.

Store at room temperature, away from heat and light; use within 1 year (or 2 years if you used jojoba oil).

TO USE: Shake well before each use. To treat foot and toenail fungus, first make sure your feet are dry. Apply a few drops to both feet, even if only one is affected. Be sure to get some of the oil between the toes and on the toenails, and massage it in thoroughly. Allow the oil to penetrate for a few minutes and then put on your socks. To treat fingernail fungus, apply a drop to each nail and massage it in thoroughly. Keep fingers away from eyes, nose, and mouth. For either treatment, repeat the application two or three times per day for several months, or until the condition abates.

Herbal Fresh Deodorant Spray

The most important action of any deodorant is to minimize the proliferation of odor-causing bacteria, and this formula, with its delightful aroma, does it amazingly well, sans synthetic fragrance and questionable ingredients. Keep a small bottle with a few cotton pads handy for when you need to freshen up a bit. It's wonderful as a foot deodorizer, too! *Safe for folks 6 years of age and older.*

ESSENTIAL OILS

16 ◆ geranium

12 ◆ rosemary (ct. verbenon)

12 ◆ tea tree

8 ◆ lemon

BASE

1 cup unflavored vodka or commercially prepared witch hazel

½ teaspoon vegetable glycerin

8-ounce plastic or dark glass spritzer bottle

TO MAKE THE SPRAY: Pour the vodka into the bottle. Add the glycerin, then the geranium, rosemary, tea tree, and lemon essential oils. Screw the top on the bottle and shake vigorously to blend. Label the bottle and allow the spray to synergize for at least 1 hour.

Store at room temperature, away from heat and light; use within 1 year.

TO USE: Shake well before each use. Spray onto clean, dry underarms and/or feet or apply with a cotton pad or cloth and rub in. Let dry before getting dressed. Follow with a natural deodorizing body powder, if desired.

Bonus uses: This formula doubles as an astringent and mild antiseptic liquid cleanser for your hands, face, or entire body, for that matter (avoid the eyes, nose, and mouth). Use for impromptu cleansing when a bath or shower is not convenient. It also makes a good mosquito repellent!

The Top 11 Essentials

MAKES 8 OUNCES (240 ML)

Lavender

(Lavandula angustifolia)

This is my absolute favorite herb! Entire books have been written about the aromatic and medicinal properties of lavender. It has a well-established tradition as a folk remedy, and its delicate old-fashioned floral scent is familiar to almost everyone. Lavender derives its name from the Latin *lavare*, meaning "to wash," as it has been used to scent baths, cosmetic waters, and natural deodorants since Roman times. The dried flowers were carried by many people during the Middle Ages because they were thought to ward off bubonic plague and other diseases. Lavender sachets are used to scent clothing drawers and bed linens, as well as to keep fiber-munching moths at bay. It's a terrific insect repellent in general. Additionally, lavender tea and tincture are traditional remedies for indigestion, colic, festering wounds, worms, sore throat, headaches, and nervous exhaustion.

Lavender essential oil appears in myriad formulas simply because it's one of the most versatile essential oils produced today, not to mention its consistent availability and affordability. It's a complete medicine chest unto itself, and it is so safe and gentle that it may be used "neat" (undiluted).

How do I integrate lavender essential oil into my life? I carry a small bottle of it with me at all times, and I use it for treating minor to moderate burns, sunburn, cuts and scrapes, insect bites and stings, rashes, muscle aches, spasmodic cramps, blemishes, bruises, tension headaches, cold and flu symptoms, nervousness and anxiety, and insomnia. In my younger days, I applied a lavender compress to my abdomen to relieve menstrual cramps and added it to my shampoo and conditioner (24 drops in an 8-ounce bottle) to keep lice and other bugs at bay.

There are so many other uses for lavender: It is truly a miraculous flower with amazing powers.

PSYCHOLOGICAL BENEFITS: Lavender is said to balance the central nervous system. Whether inhaled or topically applied, it creates calm out of chaos, harmonizing the mind, body, and spirit. It allays nervous tension, eases stress and anxiety, quells anger, lifts depression, and is a relaxing, calming aid for women suffering from emotional upheavals during PMS and menopause.

SAFETY DATA: Generally considered nontoxic, nonirritating, and nonsensitizing. Adverse reactions are extremely rare, but people with extremely low blood pressure should avoid it.

FROM HERB TO OIL

Both the pale green leaves and dusty-violet flowers of this evergreen woody shrub are highly aromatic. Indigenous to the Mediterranean and now cultivated all over the world, *Lavandula angustifolia* is the most commonly used species of true lavender.

The essential oil is steam-distilled from the flowering tops and aromatic leaves harvested before the buds open. The colorless to pale yellow liquid has a softly sweet, herbaceous, floral aroma with a woody-green undertone.

ESSENTIAL PROPERTIES

Lends aid and comfort for practically every ailment and condition, physical and emotional; extremely calming, soothing, and cooling; sedative; strongly anti-inflammatory and antibacterial; skin cell regenerator/wound healer bar none; valuable insect repellent

Lavender Lover's Bath Salts

For the lavender lover, there's nothing like a relaxing, skin-pampering bath deeply fragranced with old-fashioned lavender. This bath will soothe a tired, achy body, swollen joints, and strained muscles. It's a great way to unwind after a stress-filled day. Follow up with a head-to-toe slathering of a therapeutic lavender body cream or Lavender Lover's Massage Oil (page 70), then slip into your favorite pajamas and some cozy socks. You'll sleep like a baby. *Safe for folks 12 years of age and older.*

ESSENTIAL OIL
15 ◆ lavender

BASE
1 cup Epsom salt or sea salt

½ cup baking soda

TO MAKE THE BATH SALTS: Combine the Epsom salt and baking soda in a medium bowl and mix well. Add the lavender essential oil and stir well to combine.

TO USE: Close the bathroom door so that you capture the soothing vapors. Fill the tub with warm water. Add the bath salts to the tub and swish with your hands to thoroughly disperse the essential oil. Step in and soak for 20 to 30 minutes. Ahhh . . .

Lovely for Little Ones, Too

A lavender salt bath gently calms irritable or hyperactive children — it's guaranteed to take their energy down a few notches, leaving them with a more tranquil demeanor. For children from 6 to 11 years old, reduce the lavender essential oil to 10 drops and the salt to ½ cup, and leave the baking soda at ½ cup. For children from 2 to 5 years old, use only 5 drops of lavender essential oil, ¼ cup of salt, and ¼ cup of baking soda. For babies, use 2 or 3 drops of essential oil, 2 tablespoons of salt, and 2 tablespoons of baking soda.

Lavender Lover's Serenity Mist

This floral mist will gently guide you to that easygoing, unruffled state of mind where you feel relaxed, tranquil, and serene. Spritz it wherever you need a bit of calming essence — bedrooms, playrooms, the kitchen, or your car. You can even use it as an aromatic body mist. It's absolutely heavenly.

ESSENTIAL OIL
20–30 ◆ lavender

BASE
¼ cup water

¼ cup unflavored vodka

4-ounce plastic or dark glass spritzer bottle

TO MAKE THE SPRAY: Pour the water and vodka into the bottle, then add the lavender essential oil. Screw the top on the bottle and shake vigorously to blend. Label the bottle.

Store at room temperature, away from heat and light; use within 1 year.

TO USE: Shake well before using, and mist as desired.

Bonus uses: Lavender is a gentle yet potent antiseptic. I often spritz this blend throughout the house during cold and flu season. I also use it to clean my kitchen and bathroom countertops, and I keep a small bottle in my purse when traveling — it makes a wonderful hand sanitizer.

My Antianxiety Remedy

Lavender is definitely my go-to essential oil in times of stress and anxiety. It's pure therapy in a bottle! To receive lavender's calming, soothing effects, simply open the bottle and inhale several times directly over it, or place one or two drops on your palm, rub your palms together to warm the oil, cup your hands over your nose and mouth, close your eyes, and inhale deeply for a few minutes. Try it, won't you? A more relaxed demeanor awaits . . .

MAKES 4 OUNCES (120 ML)

The Top 11 Essentials

69

Lavender Lover's Massage Oil

This must-have skin-nourishing, restorative oil is quick and easy to make. It's incredibly soothing to body, mind, and spirit. And of course it smells sublime! *Safe for folks 12 years of age and older.*

ESSENTIAL OIL

40 ◆ lavender

BASE

½ cup almond, sunflower, or jojoba oil

1 400 IU vitamin E oil capsule (optional, but it adds skin-nourishing and antioxidant properties)

4-ounce plastic squeeze bottle or dark glass bottle with a pump or dropper top

TO MAKE THE OIL: Combine the lavender essential oil, your base oil of choice, and the vitamin E oil (if desired) in the bottle. Screw the top on the bottle and shake vigorously for 2 minutes to blend. Label the bottle.

Store at room temperature, away from heat and light; use within 1 year (or 2 years if you used jojoba oil).

TO USE: Shake well before each use. Massage directly into skin, starting with a small amount and using more as needed.

Bonus uses: This blend also makes a great bath oil; add 2 teaspoons to a full tub, swish to disperse, step in, and soak. It may also be used as a pampering after-bath body oil.

Soothe Them to Sleep

A lavender massage is a wonderful way to balance and relax cranky or hyper-active children; lavender's nervine properties, combined with your loving touch, will often calm them down quickly. For children from 6 to 11 years old, reduce the lavender essential oil to 30 drops. For babies and children up to 5 years old, use only 10 drops.

Aloe and Lavender "Burn Juice"

This simple and effective burn remedy relies on the dynamic duo of cooling aloe vera juice and soothing lavender essential oil to speed recovery of damaged skin tissue and reduce inflammation and pain. This is my go-to "burn juice," and I always keep a bottle of it in my refrigerator. *Safe for folks 6 years of age and older. For children ages 2 to 5, use only 40 drops of lavender essential oil. For infants and babies, use 20 drops or simply omit the essential oil altogether and use only aloe vera.*

ESSENTIAL OIL

80 ◆ lavender

BASE

1 cup commercially prepared aloe vera juice

8-ounce plastic or dark glass spritzer bottle

TO MAKE THE FORMULA: Combine the aloe vera juice and lavender essential oil in the bottle and shake vigorously to blend. Label the bottle, set it in the refrigerator, and allow the blend to synergize for at least 1 hour.

Store in the refrigerator, where it will keep for up to 6 months.

TO USE: Shake well before each use. This blend should be applied as soon as possible after the skin is burned, either by spraying it directly on the affected area or using it to soak a compress. Repeat several times per day, if desired, for up to several weeks, until the skin is completely healed.

Bonus uses: This formula provides immediate relief from the sting of sunburn and windburn, and it also calms the itch of contact dermatitis. It is excellent as a gentle toner for oily and normal skin, too.

The Top 11 Essentials

MAKES 8 OUNCES (240 ML)

Super Herbal Antibacterial Drops

With a cooling energy and powerful antiseptic, anti-inflammatory, and skin-cell-regenerating properties, this incredibly potent, yet gentle-on-the-skin blend, also helps relieve the itch that so often accompanies the healing of a wound. It has an intense "green medicine" fragrance. You can use it by the drop on any skin affliction to prevent or fight off infection. I recommend keeping a small bottle with you at all times, because you never know what your skin might encounter over the course of a day. *Safe for folks 12 years of age and older. This is an aromatherapeutically concentrated formula, so use only by the drop as directed.*

ESSENTIAL OILS

1 tablespoon lavender

25 ♦ German chamomile

25 ♦ tea tree

BASE

2½ teaspoons almond, extra-virgin olive, sunflower, or jojoba oil

1-ounce dark glass bottle with a dropper top

Bonus uses: These drops can be applied twice daily to blemishes, boils, bedsores or skin ulcers, ingrown toenails, ingrown hairs, and bug bites and stings to help soothe inflammation, reduce redness, and kill bacteria.

TO MAKE THE DROPS: Combine the lavender, chamomile, and tea tree essential oils in the bottle, then add your base oil of choice. Screw the top on the bottle and shake vigorously for 2 minutes to blend. Label the bottle and set it in a cool, dark location for 24 hours so that the oils can synergize.

Store at room temperature, away from heat and light; use within 1 year (or 2 years if you used jojoba oil).

TO USE: Cleanse the affected area with soap and water, your favorite natural antiseptic cleanser, or Aloe Disinfecting Wound Wash (page 96). Pat dry, give the antibacterial drops a good shake, then apply this formula by the drop, so that it just covers the wound. A little goes a long way. Gently tap the drops into the skin and surrounding area with a clean finger. Do this twice daily until the wound closes and begins to heal nicely.

The Top 11 Essentials

MAKES 1 OUNCE (30 ML)

40 Winks Herbal Pillow Drops

Lavender is an age-old aid for balancing the central nervous system. It promotes deep, restful sleep with nary a side effect. These highly aromatic pillow drops contain both lavender and Roman chamomile, yielding an amazingly tranquilizing yet gentle blend that will help you get some much needed shut-eye. If you regularly suffer from insomnia, these drops will be your friend! *Safe for folks 6 years of age and older. This is an aromatherapeutically concentrated formula, so use only by the drop as directed.*

ESSENTIAL OILS

1 tablespoon lavender

10 ♦ Roman chamomile

½-ounce dark glass bottle with a screw cap or orifice reducer cap

TO MAKE THE DROPS: Combine the lavender and chamomile essential oils in the bottle. Screw the top on the bottle and shake vigorously for 2 minutes to blend. Label the bottle and set it in a cool, dark location for 24 hours so that the oils can synergize.

Store at room temperature, away from heat and light; use within 2 years. Do not store the bottle with a dropper top, as the strong vapors will degrade the rubber tip. Store only with a screw cap.

TO USE: Using a dropper, place 2 to 4 drops on your pillowcase, or on a tissue or handkerchief that you'll hold in your hand or tuck under your head. Lie down, pull up the covers, and breathe deeply as you drift off into a more peaceful place.

Bonus uses: These drops work wonders to alleviate tension headaches. Apply a drop to each temple, a drop behind each ear, and two drops to the nape of your neck. Place 2 drops on your palms and rub your palms together to warm the oil, then lie down with your eyes closed, place your palms over your mouth and nose, and breathe deeply of the vapors for 20 minutes.

To take the edge off of menstrual cramps, dilute 12 drops into 1 teaspoon of castor oil (or your favorite base oil) and massage this blend into your abdomen. Cover with a light cloth and top with a hot water bottle or heating pad. Lie down and rest for 30 minutes.

To help relieve leg cramps, dilute 12 drops into 1 to 2 teaspoons of your favorite base oil and massage into the affected muscles. For children 6 to 11 years old, reduce the essential oil to 6 drops; for children 2 to 5 years old, use 3 drops; for children under 2 years old, use 1 or 2 drops.

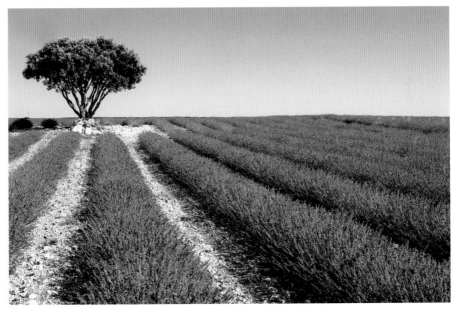

A whole field of lavender — imagine how wonderful it must smell!

Super Blister Barrier and Treatment Oil

Extra thick and with incredible staying power, this formula serves as an effective blister preventive barrier for the feet and a remedial treatment for both feet and hands once blisters have formed. It conditions skin, helps heal damaged tissue, acts as a mild astringent, reduces inflammation, and prevents infection. *Safe for folks 12 years of age and older. For children ages 6 to 11, reduce the essential oils by half.*

ESSENTIAL OILS
15 ◆ lavender

3 ◆ lemon

BASE
1 tablespoon castor oil

1 tablespoon jojoba oil

1-ounce dark glass bottle with a dropper top

TO MAKE THE OIL: Combine the lavender and lemon essential oils in the bottle, then add the castor and jojoba oils. Screw the top on the bottle and shake vigorously for 2 minutes to blend. Label the bottle and set it in a cool, dark location for 24 hours so that the oils can synergize.

Store at room temperature, away from heat and light; use within 1 year.

TO USE: Shake well before each use. To prevent blisters from forming on your feet, apply a thin coating to dry feet prior to doing any physical activity, then don socks (and make sure your footwear fits properly). To treat new blisters, apply 1 or 2 drops of this oil to each blister. Use twice daily or as desired.

Bonus uses: Apply 1 drop per nail and massage thoroughly to condition dry fingernails and cuticles and encourage growth. Omit the essential oils and it can be used as a thick lip gloss!

Lemon

Citrus limon

Delightfully refreshing and invigorating, lemons have long been regarded as something of a cure-all, especially with regard to infectious illnesses, as they are high in bioavailable vitamin C. They also deliver moderate amounts of potassium, folic acid, and capillary-strengthening flavonoids. Both the juice and peel have been used to reduce fever in cases of malaria and typhoid, prevent colds, moderate acidic disorders such as rheumatism and arthritis, and treat dysentery and liver congestion.

I've had a longtime love affair with lemon essential oil — it just gets my energy going and lifts my mood! It also tones and tightens skin tissue due to its astringent and diuretic action, being a common ingredient in formulas used to treat edema, cellulite, and bruises, as well as oily and acneic skin. Its strong antibacterial and antiviral properties help prevent and/or combat infections resulting from colds and flu, plus it aids in healing all manner of skin ailments, from minor cuts, scrapes, and insect bites to warts, boils, ulcers, and pustular eruptions.

Lemon's bright aroma freshens and cleans the air. Especially when combined with eucalyptus essential oil in a spray, it makes an invaluable air purifier during cold and flu season.

Lemon oil serves as a tonic for the circulatory system, helping to strengthen capillaries while improving sluggish blood and lymphatic flow, so I recommend it in massage oil formulations — often mixed with cypress essential oil — for those with a weak venous system, exhibiting varicose and spider veins in the legs. It's great for reviving tired, achy legs, too, especially when combined with peppermint essential oil.

PSYCHOLOGICAL BENEFITS: Lemon promotes a sunny disposition, lifting the emotions and improving states of depression, confusion, fearfulness, impurity, indecisiveness, lethargy, general debility, and that "stuck-in-the-mud" feeling. It clears mental fog and can be helpful during PMS if you're feeling blue. Like other citrus oils, it builds your sense of humor and general feeling of well-being.

SAFETY DATA: Considered nontoxic. Use in moderation and highly diluted, as it is a potential skin irritant; it may cause photosensitivity to skin exposed to sunlight and/or tanning beds within 12 hours of use.

FROM HERB TO OIL

A small evergreen tree growing to 20 feet tall with serrated, shiny, oval leaves, stiff thorns, and small, sweetly fragrant, white flowers, lemon is cultivated worldwide. Most of the essential oil is produced in Spain, Italy, and the United States, by cold expression from the outer part of the fresh peel of the ripe fruit. Steam-distilled essential oil is produced for the food/flavoring industries, but it is considered inferior for aromatherapeutic purposes.

A pale greenish-yellow liquid that turns light brownish with age, it has that familiar bright, fresh, cleansing citrus scent. Lemon essential oil has a short shelf life (as do all citrus oils), so use it within 1 year, or 2 years if you keep it refrigerated.

ESSENTIAL PROPERTIES

Very refreshing, energizing, cooling, and mentally uplifting; antidepressant; excellent anti-infectious agent, being strongly antibacterial and antiviral; cleansing and purifying; good astringent and diuretic; deodorizing; circulatory and mental stimulant

Herbal Lemon-Aid for Hands and Nails

Our hands are constantly exposed to harsh cleansers, dirt, grease, and just plain hard work. No wonder they're one of the first places on our body to show age! This mentally uplifting blend, with its base of soothing comfrey oil, is designed to condition brittle or ragged fingernails and cuticles, nurture dry hands, stimulate circulation, promote nail growth, and relieve stiffness and achiness. It also acts as an antiseptic, keeping potential infection at bay if you happen to have a nick or cut on your fingers. If you massage it into your hands and nails daily, expect to see happy, comfortable, healthy hands and nails within a couple of months. *Safe for folks 12 years of age and older. Do not apply to open wounds.*

ESSENTIAL OILS

8 ◆ lemon

8 ◆ rosemary (ct. verbenon or nonchemotype specific)

4 ◆ lavender

4 ◆ peppermint

BASE

¼ cup comfrey-infused oil (page 212)

2-ounce dark glass bottle with a dropper top

TO MAKE THE BLEND: Combine the lemon, rosemary, lavender, and peppermint essential oils in the bottle, then add the comfrey oil. Screw the top on the bottle and shake vigorously for 2 minutes to blend. Label the bottle and set it in a cool, dark location for 24 hours so that the oils can synergize.

Store at room temperature, away from heat and light; use within 1 year.

TO USE: Shake well before each use. Massage several drops into your hands and nails (whether dry or damp) once or twice daily. For best results, be consistent with this ritual. Keep hands away from eyes after application.

Lemon essential oil is often diffused therapeutically in hospitals for its antiseptic properties and to cheer up patients and staff, as well as for its amazing ability to neutralize that notorious "hospital smell."

The Top 11 Essentials

MAKES 2 OUNCES (60 ML)

Lemony-Mint Mojito Breath Spray

Imagine slightly sweet lemonade muddled with peppermint leaves . . . oh my! That's the flavor punch delivered by this super-freshening, cooling breath spray. It's guaranteed to help neutralize odor-causing bacteria and any unpleasant food flavors lingering in your mouth. Why not make several bottles? The convenient small size makes it easy to stash this blend in your purse, backpack, briefcase, gym bag, desk drawer, bathroom cabinet — almost anywhere! *Safe for folks 12 years of age and older.*

ESSENTIAL OILS

3 ◆ lemon

2 ◆ peppermint

BASE

4 teaspoons purified water

1 teaspoon vegetable glycerin

1 teaspoon unflavored vodka

1-ounce plastic or dark glass spritzer bottle

TO MAKE THE SPRAY: Combine the lemon and peppermint essential oils in the bottle, then add the water, glycerin, and vodka. Screw the top on the bottle and shake vigorously to blend. Label the bottle and allow the spray to synergize for 1 hour.

Store at room temperature, away from heat and light; use within 1 year.

TO USE: Shake the bottle immediately before each use. Spray once or twice into your mouth to cleanse and freshen your breath.

MAKES 1 OUNCE (30 ML)

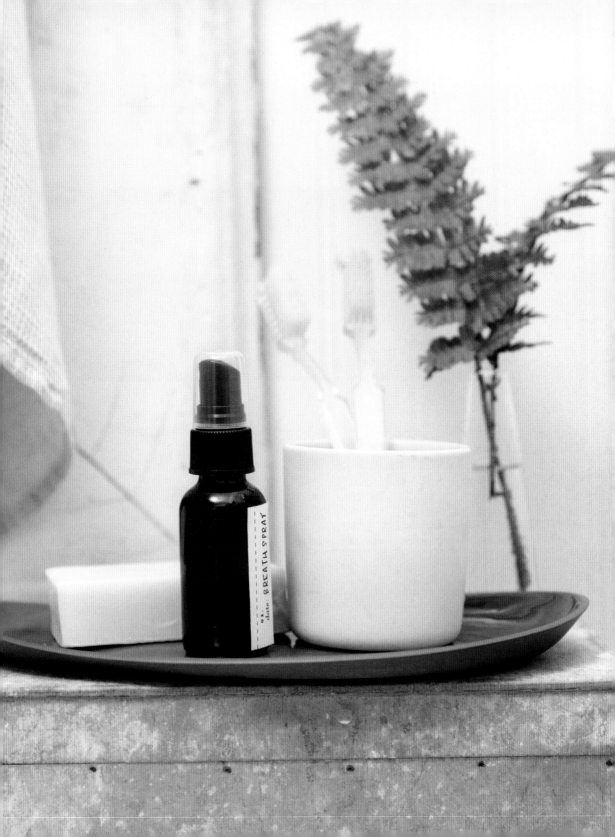

Peppermint

(Mentha piperita)

Mints have been cultivated by many cultures for thousands of years and used extensively in both Eastern and Western medicine for a variety of complaints, including indigestion, colic, flatulence, nausea, motion sickness, diarrhea, vomiting during pregnancy, headaches, toothaches, muscular cramps, and fever.

We typically think of peppermint as being cooling and refreshing, but it can also be warming, especially when used in a liniment or massage oil blend. How? Upon contact, the essential oil constricts capillaries, which leads to a bracing, chilling sensation. The body responds by dramatically increasing blood flow in the affected area, which leads to a warming sensation. This constriction-expansion of blood flow makes peppermint an excellent choice for treating poor circulation.

Menthol, peppermint's most prominent chemical component, has quite a remarkable stimulating action on the respiratory system. Peppermint oil opens the respiratory channels and is great combined with rosemary and eucalyptus essential oils for symptoms of sinus and lung congestion; it really improves oxygen uptake, helps thin mucus, and combats infection.

Peppermint also relaxes the muscles of the digestive tract and stimulates bile flow, making it a wonderfully effective remedy for many cases of digestive ailments. It is one of my favorite remedies for bad breath, indigestion, motion sickness, and nausea — it works like a charm!

Its cooling, astringent action quickly relieves hot flashes, tension headaches and migraines, and fatigued, swollen legs and feet. I add it to formulations designed to deliver pain relief to cramped muscles, stressed ligaments and tendons, and the inflammation of rheumatoid arthritis and gout.

PSYCHOLOGICAL BENEFITS: As a mental stimulant, peppermint promotes clarity of thought and encourages positivity. It aids the mind in breaking free from an emotionally "stuck" pattern, while strengthening resolve and courage. It counters mental fogginess, confusion, lack of focus, depression, general debility, lethargy, nervous exhaustion, and anxiety.

SAFETY DATA: Generally considered nontoxic and nonirritating (except in concentration); may cause sensitization in some individuals due to the menthol concentration. Use in moderation. Avoid if pregnant or breastfeeding. Use with caution on or near the face of very young children, as it can be a mucous membrane irritant, although the risk is low. Peppermint essential oil is *not* compatible with homeopathic treatment.

FROM HERB TO OIL

Peppermint, an intensely fragrant perennial herb with leafy stems and lilac-colored flowers, is easily propagated. It has naturalized in North America, Europe, and Australia and is cultivated worldwide. The essential oil is primarily produced in the United States by steam distillation of the fresh flowering tops and leaves. It is a pale yellow or greenish liquid with a highly penetrating, refreshing, sometimes grassy-sweet odor. It can become quite viscous when exposed to cold temperatures.

ESSENTIAL PROPERTIES

Both cooling and warming, depending on how it is used; energizing and refreshing; circulatory and cognitive stimulant; analgesic, antibacterial, and astringent; superb carminative and digestive aid; deodorizing; valuable insect repellent and parasiticide, useful in combating scabies, lice, and ringworm

Lini-Mint Foot Chiller

My country-living grandfather used to tell me that the fastest way to cool off and reenergize on a hot day was to immerse your hot, sweaty feet in an icy cold creek. "Literally pulls the heat right out of you," he'd say. If you lack an invigorating creek, refreshing herbal relief is a quick spray away with this simple formula. Vodka and peppermint essential oil form a menthol-infused liniment of moderate intensity, with a cool to cold energy that evaporates rapidly, removing heat along with sweat and odor, leaving you feeling footloose and fancy-free.

It's perfect for teens, or anyone, with odoriferous "dogs!" I recommend stashing a small bottle in your gym bag to use as a post-workout foot refresher, especially if there's no time to shower. It'll put some spring back in your step! *Safe for folks 2 years of age and older.*

ESSENTIAL OIL
30 ◗ peppermint

BASE
1 cup unflavored vodka

½ teaspoon vegetable glycerin

8-ounce plastic or dark glass spritzer bottle

TO MAKE THE SPRAY: Combine the vodka, glycerin, and peppermint essential oil in the bottle. Screw on the cap and shake vigorously to blend. Label the bottle.

Store at room temperature, away from heat and light; use within 1 year. No refrigeration is required, but chilling the formula makes it even more refreshing and invigorating!

TO USE: Shake well before each use. Spray on bare feet whenever they're feeling hot or in need of refreshment. Allow your feet to air-dry.

Bonus use: This spray doubles as a superior room freshener. Simply spritz into the air a few times and say good-bye to staleness and odor.

Peppermint Nausea Relief

Nausea . . . that awful queasiness in the pit of your stomach that often produces the urge to vomit . . . yuck! Whatever the cause, peppermint, a well-known carminative (digestive aid), is a go-to herb for easing this distressing ailment. This double-whammy recipe combines a soothing beverage with calming inhalation for quick, convenient, aromatically pleasing relief!

BEVERAGE

1 cup warm or cold water, as preferred

The juice of half a lime or lemon

1 teaspoon of raw honey

1 ♦ of peppermint

A pinch of sea salt

Mix thoroughly, then sip very slowly. Repeat up to three times per day.

Do not serve this beverage to children under 12 years of age.

INHALATION

1 ♦ peppermint

1 ♦ lavender or ginger (optional, but either one can enhance the antinausea properties and also soften the sharp aromatic edge of peppermint if you find it too strong)

TO USE: Place the drop of peppermint essential oil and the lavender or ginger essential oil (if desired) in your palm and rub both palms together to warm the oil. Immediately cup your hands over your nose and mouth and inhale deeply for 15 to 30 seconds. Avoid direct contact with the eyes, nose, and mouth. Repeat several times.

Safe for folks 6 years of age and older. For children ages 2 to 5, apply the essential oils to a facial tissue, not to the child's palms.

Foot Soak for Headache Relief

Want a quick and utterly simple remedy for a tension headache? Take a load off and soak your feet in cold water for a spell. It draws blood from your head, easing the heat and muscular tightness that are causing your headache. With the addition of peppermint, plus lavender or geranium essential oil, to your foot soak, your whole body will receive energetically balancing and cooling aromatherapeutic benefits, while you soften and deodorize your poor tired feet. *Safe for folks 6 years of age and older.*

ESSENTIAL OILS
5 ● lavender or geranium

3 ● peppermint

BASE
2 teaspoons vegetable glycerin

TO MAKE THE SOAK: Combine the glycerin with the essential oils in a small bowl, such as a custard cup, and stir thoroughly to mix.

TO USE: Pour the essential oil blend into a foot tub with enough very cold water (and maybe a few ice cubes) to cover your feet and ankles. Swish with your feet to blend. Soak your feet for 10 to 15 minutes, with your eyes closed, while breathing deeply and regularly. Then briskly dry your feet with a thick, rough towel and follow with an application of a peppermint foot lotion or your favorite moisturizer. You feel a lot better now, don't you?

Rosemary

(Rosmarinus officinalis)

Rosemary is one of the earliest known plants to be used in many cultures for medicine, skin and hair care, food, purification, incense, and magic. It is an herbal ally whose scent I find absolutely alluring, and I utilize some form of it daily — in tea, as an infused oil or essential oil in topical remedies, or as a culinary seasoning. Everyone should have a rosemary plant growing in their garden or in their home.

The strongly aromatic leaves are highly valued for their antiseptic properties. In times past they were burned as a fumigant during epidemics to protect against plague and infectious illness, and French hospitals still utilized this practice into the twentieth century.

Rosemary essential oil is a classic ingredient in shampoo and conditioning formulations to enhance hair growth and shine, balance an oily scalp, and control dandruff, as it tones, tightens, and astringes skin tissue. It is also recommended to combat lice, scabies, and ringworm.

Rosemary's warming, analgesic action makes it helpful in the treatment of cold hands and feet, arthritis, rheumatism, and gout, especially in cases where symptoms are worse in cold weather. Stiff, sore, inflamed muscles, sprains, and strains respond quickly to rosemary, making it a classic ingredient in post-workout blends. On the flip side, rosemary oil is also used to enhance circulation and warmth in muscles prior to sporting activities, in an effort to minimize injury.

In my reflexology practice I often see clients with edema of the lower legs and feet. Rosemary is one of the primary essential oils I use to aid in lymphatic drainage, as it is of much benefit to relieve conditions of swelling, fatigue, achiness, and heaviness.

PSYCHOLOGICAL BENEFITS: As a powerful mental stimulant, rosemary promotes clarity of thought, creativity, perception, and confidence. It counters mental fatigue, amnesia, confusion, lack of focus, general debility, lethargy, and anxiety. Its sharp fragrance is uplifting in times of depression, grief, emotional shock, dark thoughts, nightmares, apathy, and the premenstrual blues. It can help you move forward from past relationship hurts, enabling you to more comfortably form close, trusting emotional bonds once again.

SAFETY DATA: *R. officinalis* and *R. officinalis* ct. cineole are considered nontoxic, generally nonirritating, and nonsensitizing (except in concentration). They may cause dermatitis in those with sensitive skin. *R. officinalis* ct. verbenon is the most gentle of the rosemary essential oils and is generally considered safe, gentle, and nonirritating.

Avoid *all* varieties of rosemary essential oil if you are pregnant. Avoid using *R. officinalis* ct. cineole and nonchemotype-specific *R. officinalis* on or near the face of children under the age of 10, as it is considered too stimulating to the central nervous system and may cause breathing difficulties.

Known as the herb of remembrance, rosemary has long been valued for improving sluggish circulation, oxygenating the brain, and enhancing memory. Greek and Roman students wore garlands of rosemary about their heads while studying for examinations. You can experience rosemary's brain-boosting effects much more easily by placing a drop or two onto a tissue and inhaling it while you work.

FROM HERB TO OIL

Rosemary is a shrubby evergreen bush with needle-shaped, slightly resinous, leathery leaves and lavender-blue, white, or pale pink flowers. The entire plant is strongly aromatic. *Rosmarinus* means "dew of the sea," a nod to this native Mediterranean herb's affinity for seaside environs. Rosemary is now cultivated in many regions around the world, but the principal oil-producing countries are France, Spain, Tunisia, and Morocco. The best-quality oil is steam-distilled from the fresh flowering tops and leaves.

The essential oil is a colorless or pale yellow liquid with a strong, sharp minty-herbaceous scent and a woody-balsamic undertone. Poor-quality oils have a more potent camphorous note.

R. officinalis is the most widely available variety of rosemary essential oil. I often prefer *R. officinalis* ct. cineole, which has a similar aroma, in blends to ease headaches, help heal respiratory infections, or rid the lungs of "stuck" mucus. It also works wonders when I need an amped-up energizing and circulation-stimulating effect. If ct. cineole is unavailable, then nonchemotype-specific rosemary essential oil may be used instead.

The essential oil of *R. officinalis* ct. verbenon has a milder, slightly lemony aroma, and it is less stimulating and amazingly gentle. It's wonderfully healing and rejuvenating for all skin types, it is a powerful antiseptic, and its ability to thin mucus is virtually unequalled by other essential oils. When you need rosemary's power with a gentler nature, choose this one.

ESSENTIAL PROPERTIES

Strong antibacterial with an affinity for the respiratory system; analgesic; circulatory and cognitive stimulant, wonderful for enhancing concentration and focus; antidepressant; energizing and warming; deodorizing; speeds skin cell regeneration; superb wound healer; traditional hair and scalp oil; valuable insect repellent and parasiticide

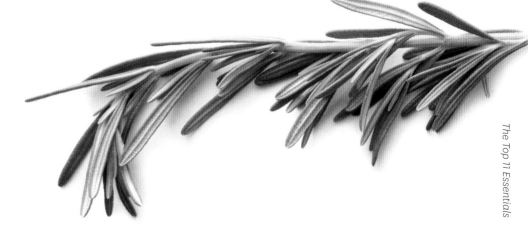

The Top 11 Essentials

Tension Headache Roll-On Remedy

Tension headaches, often brought on by excessive stress, are the most common type of headache. Though not as severe as a migraine, the pain is truly uncomfortable and annoying. This handy, aromatic roll-on formula is recommended for direct spot treatment to the areas on your head and neck that ache, throb, and feel constricted. If applied immediately at the onset of a headache, it may deliver a preemptive strike, warding off any further development of the headache. *Safe for folks 12 years of age and older. This is an aromatherapeutically concentrated formula, so use only as directed.*

ESSENTIAL OILS

- 6 ◆ rosemary (ct. cineole or nonchemotype specific)
- 4 ◆ lavender
- 4 ◆ Roman chamomile
- 2 ◆ peppermint

BASE

- 2 teaspoons jojoba or fractionated coconut oil
- 10 ml roller-ball applicator bottle

TO MAKE THE REMEDY: Combine the rosemary, lavender, chamomile, and peppermint essential oils in the bottle, then add your base oil of choice. Cap and shake vigorously for 2 minutes. Label the bottle and set it in a cool, dark location for 24 hours so that the oils can synergize.

Store at room temperature, away from heat and light; use within 2 years.

TO USE: Shake well before each use. When you feel a tension headache coming on, roll a little oil onto each temple, the nape of the neck, and the forehead region. Massage in well. Next, roll some onto one palm, rub your palms together to warm the oil, then cup your hands over your mouth and nose, close your eyes, and inhale the vapors. Breathe slowly and deeply for a few minutes. Avoid direct contact with the eyes, nose, and mouth. Repeat several times throughout the day, as needed, until you feel better.

Energize Me!

This pleasingly sharp blend of ultra-stimulating essential oils opens the sinus and respiratory channels, inviting a rush of fresh, energizing oxygen to your brain and lungs. Take a whiff first thing in the morning to help you wake up and motivate you to take on the day's tasks, or use it in the afternoon to keep production levels high at work. It makes a wonderful diffuser blend to enliven the home or office environment, or to use in teenagers' rooms while they're doing homework. *Safe for folks 12 years of age and older. This is an aromatherapeutically concentrated formula, so use only by the drop as directed.*

ESSENTIAL OILS

60 ◆ rosemary (ct. verbenon or nonchemotype specific)

50 ◆ peppermint

40 ◆ eucalyptus (species *globulus*, *radiata*, or *smithii*)

¼-ounce dark glass bottle with a screw cap or orifice reducer cap

Bonus uses: Containing decongestant, respiratory-disinfecting, and antiviral properties, this blend is recommended for use in a diffuser for anyone suffering from sinus or chest congestion, bronchial infections, a bad cold, or the flu. Follow the manufacturer's directions for your particular brand of essential oil diffuser or nebulizer, and use the appropriate number of drops.

TO MAKE THE BLEND: Combine the rosemary, peppermint, and eucalyptus essential oils in the bottle. Screw the top on the bottle and shake vigorously for 2 minutes to blend. Label the bottle and set it in a cool, dark location for 24 hours so that the oils can synergize.

Store at room temperature, away from heat and light; use within 2 years. Do not store the bottle with a dropper top, as the strong vapors will degrade the rubber tip. Store only with a screw cap.

TO USE: Shake well before using. Place only 1 or 2 drops in your palm, rub both palms together to warm the oil, cup your hands over your nose and mouth, and inhale deeply for 15 to 30 seconds. Avoid direct contact with the eyes, nose, and mouth. Repeat two or three times per day, if needed.

Caution: If you suffer from asthma, this formulation may be too stimulating. Avoid completely if you are having an asthma attack.

The Top 11 Essentials

Rosemary Remembrance Balm

Amazingly refreshing, stimulating, uplifting, rejuvenating, and clarifying, this balm is just the thing to awaken your brain and help you recall and retain what you seem to have forgotten! If you resonate with rosemary as much I do, you'll appreciate this balm. *Safe for folks 12 years of age and older.*

ESSENTIAL OIL

60 ● rosemary (ct. verbenon or nonchemotype specific)

BASE

7 tablespoons almond, jojoba, extra-virgin olive, or sunflower oil

1–2 tablespoons beeswax (depending on how firm a balm you want)

4-ounce dark glass or plastic jar

TO MAKE THE BALM: Combine your base oil of choice and the beeswax in a small saucepan over low heat, or in a double boiler, and warm until the beeswax is just melted. Remove from the heat and allow to cool for 5 minutes, stirring a few times. Add the rosemary essential oil and stir again to thoroughly blend. Slowly pour the liquid balm into the jar. Cap immediately and label. Set aside for 30 minutes to thicken.

Store at room temperature, away from heat and light; use within 1 year (or 2 years if you used jojoba oil).

TO USE: For memory enhancement, apply a little dab of this balm to your temples, the nape of your neck, the base of your throat, and behind each ear up to three times daily. Breathe deeply of the invigorating vapors.

Bonus uses: This balm also aids in healing dry, cracked skin on the feet, hands, nails, shins, elbows, and knees. I use it occasionally to condition the ends of my very dry hair and as a blister balm when I'm hiking. It even helps heal oozing poison plant rashes and dermatitis. If you have a stuffy head, massage a dab on your chest, on your neck, and under your nose. This is good stuff!

Invigorating Daily Body Wash

Here's a gentle body wash with an eye-opening, ultra-fresh scent guaranteed to start your day on a zippy note! This combination of skin-nurturing, moisturizing ingredients produces a creamy lather that leaves skin feeling silky soft and smooth. *Safe for use by folks 12 years of age and older.*

ESSENTIAL OILS
14 ◊ rosemary (ct. verbenon or nonchemotype specific)

10 ◊ peppermint

6 ◊ lemon

BASE
4 tablespoons unscented liquid castile soap

2 tablespoons plus 2 teaspoons commercially prepared aloe vera juice

1 tablespoon almond, jojoba, or sunflower oil

1 teaspoon vegetable glycerin

4-ounce plastic pump or squeeze bottle

TO MAKE THE WASH: Combine the castile soap, aloe vera juice, your base oil of choice, and vegetable glycerin in a small bowl and mix well. Add the rosemary, peppermint, and lemon essential oils and gently stir until well blended. Pour into the bottle. Screw on the cap and shake vigorously for approximately 20 seconds. Label the bottle and allow the blend to synergize for 1 hour.

Store in the shower, where it will keep for up to 2 months, and then make a fresh batch.

TO USE: Shake well before each use. Apply as a body wash using your hands, a washcloth, or a sponge, working the blend into a light, creamy lather. Rinse.

Bonus use: This formula makes a wonderful shaving product for both men and women.

The Top 11 Essentials

MAKES 4 OUNCES (120 ML)

Tea Tree

(Melaleuca alternifolia)

Tea tree has a very long history of use by the Australian Aboriginal people for treatment of infected wounds and skin problems. Tea tree essential oil, however, is a relatively new addition to aromatherapy. It is closely related to cajeput (*M. cajuputi*) and niaouli (*M. quinquenervia*), with which it shares many of the same properties, but tea tree is considered more powerful. The oil is quite unusual in that it is effective against all three varieties of infectious organisms: viruses, bacteria, and fungi. As a potent immune stimulant, it also increases the body's ability to respond when threatened by any of these organisms. No wonder it is called "nature's first aid tree"!

This is one of the few oils that can be used "neat" or undiluted, so it is a convenient spot treatment for herpes lesions, acne blemishes, insect bites and stings, warts, corns, athlete's foot, fungal nails, cuts and scrapes, boils, skin ulcers, localized rashes, burns, toothache, and puncture wounds. Powerful yet gentle, tea tree essential oil is a must-have for your home medicine cabinet.

For women, tea tree oil can deliver blessed relief from the itching and burning that accompany vaginitis and vaginal yeast infections. A few drops combined with vinegar and water makes a comforting, cleansing douche. Men can add it to a sitz bath to help eradicate jock itch.

Respiratory congestion as well as deep-seated infections, such as bronchitis, sinusitis, rhinitis, pneumonia, and pertussis (whooping cough), respond favorably to tea tree's healing strength.

PSYCHOLOGICAL BENEFITS: The scent is mentally fortifying, strengthening, revitalizing, cleansing, and purifying. It is especially beneficial in cases of general debility, nervous exhaustion, and shock following traumatic events or surgery.

SAFETY DATA: Nontoxic and nonirritating; potentially sensitizing in some individuals if used undiluted.

Soldiers stationed in the tropics during World War II used tea tree essential oil to treat wounds.

FROM HERB TO OIL

Native to Australia and growing to a height of approximately 22 feet, tea tree is one of the smallest of the myrtle family. It has needle-like leaves similar to cypress and bears fluffy, creamy-white masses of flowers from spring to early summer. Tea tree is commercially cultivated in Australia, Tasmania, and Kenya. The essential oil is produced by steam distillation of the leaves and twigs. Light yellowish-green or colorless, it has a strong, fresh medicinal odor with hints of turpentine.

ESSENTIAL PROPERTIES

A medicine chest in a bottle: a broad-spectrum antibacterial, antifungal, and antiviral; gentle to the skin and amazingly effective against a wide range of ailments, especially infections of the skin, respiratory tract, and mouth; immunostimulant; energizing; cooling; effective against lice, scabies, and ringworm

Aloe Disinfecting Wound Wash

This super-easy wound wash should be in everyone's medicine cabinet. It rinses away dirt and debris while keeping microbes at bay, speeding the healing process. This remedy can also be used as a daily disinfectant while the wound is healing. Take a small bottle with you when hiking or camping for on-the-spot treatment. *Safe for folks 6 years of age and older.*

ESSENTIAL OILS

50 ◆ lavender

50 ◆ tea tree

BASE

1 cup commercially prepared aloe vera juice

1 cup unflavored vodka

16-ounce plastic squeeze bottle

TO MAKE THE WASH: Combine the lavender and tea tree essential oils in the bottle, then add the aloe vera juice and vodka. Screw the top on the bottle and shake vigorously for 2 minutes to blend. Label the bottle and set it in a cool, dark location for 24 hours so that the formula can synergize.

Store at room temperature, away from heat and light; use within 6 months.

TO USE: Shake well before each use. If possible, first clean the cut or scrape using mild soap and water. Then squirt the liniment directly over the affected area, thoroughly soaking the injury. Pat dry, then apply Stephanie's Essential Heal-All Oil (page 50) or your favorite wound-healing ointment or salve. Fasten a sterile nonstick pad over the injury, if needed. Apply the formula to the wound twice daily until it heals. This is especially recommended if the wound is presenting infection or is slow to heal.

Bonus use: This wash works wonderfully well as a spot treatment for acne blemishes and bug bites and stings.

Vinegar and Tea Tree Vaginitis Relief

A delicate subject, I realize, but all women should have on hand the natural ingredients needed to help remedy vaginitis, or inflammation of vaginal tissue, an irritating, uncomfortable condition often accompanied by external itching, burning upon urination, minor discharge, and odor. This douche aids in reestablishing the naturally acidic pH level in the vagina and leaves behind a fresh, healthy feeling. It's helpful as a gentle treatment for minor to moderate yeast infections, too.

ESSENTIAL OIL

10 ◆ tea tree

BASE

7½ cups warm water, preferably purified and nonchlorinated

½ cup apple cider vinegar (preferably organic and unpasteurized)

TO MAKE THE BLEND: Combine all ingredients in a 2-quart douche bag and screw in the stopper.

TO USE: Give the bag a good shake immediately before use. Proceed as you would normally when douching. See your health-care provider if symptoms persist. Thoroughly wash the bag, hose, and tip with hot soapy water after use.

EO Extra: Tea Tree

For mouth and throat care, tea tree oil is ultra-effective against the germs that cause bad breath, gingivitis, and ulcers, and when used as a gargle, it can relieve the pain and inflammation of an infected sore throat, laryngitis, and irritation resulting from thrush. To use, add 1 drop of tea tree essential oil to 1 tablespoon of warm water. Stir vigorously and immediately gargle for at least 30 seconds (or as long as possible), then spit out in the sink. Repeat up to three times per day. Recommended for folks 12 years of age and older.

The Top 11 Essentials

MAKES ENOUGH FOR 1 TREATMENT

Herpes Relief Drops

A contagious viral infection, *Herpes simplex* manifests around the mouth (as cold sores or fever blisters) or the genitals. *H. zoster*, also known as shingles, is caused by the chickenpox virus and is quite painful. Both strains can lie dormant in the nervous system for years; eruptions are often triggered by a heavy load of stress. This herbal formula offers effective antiseptic, antiviral, circulation-stimulating, and skin-conditioning properties and feels nice and cool when applied to burning, itching herpes lesions. The aroma is unusual but pleasant, and not overly medicinal. *Safe for folks 12 years of age and older. This is an aroma-therapeutically concentrated formula, so use only by the drop as directed.*

ESSENTIAL OILS
- 6 ◆ eucalyptus (species *globulus*, *radiata*, or *smithii*)
- 6 ◆ tea tree
- 2 ◆ geranium
- 2 ◆ lavender
- 2 ◆ peppermint

BASE
- 2 tablespoons tamanu oil
- 1-ounce dark glass bottle with a dropper top

TO MAKE THE DROPS: Combine the eucalyptus, tea tree, geranium, lavender, and peppermint essential oils in the bottle, then add the tamanu oil. Screw the top on the bottle and shake vigorously for 2 minutes to blend. Label the bottle and set it in a cool, dark location for 24 hours so that the oils can synergize.

Store at room temperature, away from heat and light; use within 1 year.

TO USE: Shake well prior to each use. Apply to affected area up to three times per day. If a burning or stinging sensation develops, immediately remove product from the area with a tissue and a small amount of vegetable oil.

Acne-Clear Spot Treatment

This potent antimicrobial and anti-inflammatory facial blend is formulated to help clear blemishes, acne, and minor skin infections. It inhibits subsurface bacterial growth, cleans pores, and restores the health of underlying tissue. *Safe for folks 12 years of age and older. This is an aromatherapeutically concentrated formula, so use only as directed.*

ESSENTIAL OILS
- 6 ◆ tea tree
- 4 ◆ lavender
- 3 ◆ rosemary (ct. verbenon)
- 2 ◆ thyme (ct. linalool)
- 1 ◆ German chamomile

BASE
- 2 teaspoons unflavored vodka
- 10 ml roller-ball applicator bottle

TO MAKE THE BLEND: Combine the tea tree, lavender, rosemary, thyme, and chamomile essential oils in the bottle, then add the vodka. Cap and shake vigorously for 2 minutes. Label the bottle and set it in a cool, dark location for 24 hours so that the oils can synergize.

Store at room temperature, away from heat and light; use within 2 years.

TO USE: Shake well prior to each use. Apply directly on affected area two or three times per day, and especially before going to sleep. *Do not* apply over your entire face, as the alcohol base is too drying for any unaffected skin tissue, and the essential oil concentration is much too strong for more than spot-treatment coverage.

Quick and "Neat" Insect Bite and Sting Relief

Tea tree and lavender can be safely applied to the skin "neat" or undiluted. To gain quick relief from bites and stings, apply a drop of either essential oil directly to the affected area up to three times per day until the discomfort has subsided. *Always* keep a small bottle of these essential oils in your medicine cabinet. Between the two, they can treat and reduce the discomfort of almost any minor malady!

The Top 11 Essentials

MAKES 10 ML

Thyme

(Thymus vulgaris)

Pleasingly aromatic thyme was frequently used in medicine, cosmetics, food, perfume, incense, and embalming rituals by the ancient Greeks, Egyptians, and Romans, and it has a long history of use as a medicinal plant in the Western herbal apothecary. Whether utilized as a tea, tincture, syrup, or essential oil, thyme's main arenas of remediation have been and still are digestive complaints, respiratory problems, circulatory disorders, muscle and joint discomforts, and the prevention and treatment of infection.

I primarily use thyme essential oil in blends intended to fend off and/or combat cold and flu symptoms. I also use it in air purification spritzers, topically, and in inhalation sticks. Thyme is mighty medicine against infectious nasties!

PSYCHOLOGICAL BENEFITS: Thyme essential oil can be both stimulating and relaxing to the mind, so it tends to regulate the psyche as needed. The uplifting, clarifying, refreshing scent instills courage, fortifies the spirit, and strengthens the will, while dispelling fear, mental instability, melancholy, nightmares, and nervous exhaustion.

SAFETY DATA: *T. vulgaris* and *T. vulgaris* ct. thymol are dermal and mucous membrane irritants and should be used in moderation and highly diluted. Avoid if you are pregnant or breastfeeding. Topical application (and ingestion) is best avoided if you are using anticoagulants, following major surgery, or if you suffer from peptic ulcer, hemophilia, or another bleeding disorder.

T. vulgaris ct. linalool is generally nonirritating and nontoxic; it is gentler on the skin and safe to use during pregnancy/lactation and with children, the elderly, and those with a weakened constitution.

FROM HERB TO OIL

Common garden thyme is the cultivated form of wild thyme (*T. serpyllum*), which derives its name from its serpent-like growth. Native to Spain and the Mediterranean region, it has spread throughout the world, but the main oil-producing countries are France, Hungary, Morocco, Turkey, and Spain. Steam distillation of the fresh or partially dried leaves and flowering tops produces several types of essential oil.

T. vulgaris, often referred to as common thyme or red thyme, has a scent that can be described as medicinal, warm-herbaceous, somewhat spicy, and slightly sweet. With high levels of the constituent thymol it — especially the variety *T. vulgaris* ct. thymol — demands respect, as it can be quite irritating if not heavily diluted. Thymol relieves lung congestion and is effective against gingivitis and bad breath.

T. vulgaris ct. linalool, commonly known as sweet thyme or mild thyme, yields a clear, pale yellow essential oil that has a sweeter, softer antiseptic aroma. It is considerably milder than the other thyme varieties. When you need thyme's remedial power yet desire a gentler, cooler, less irritating effect, this is the one to choose.

ESSENTIAL PROPERTIES

One of the most anti-infectious of all oils and an ideal choice to use against respiratory, mouth, and skin infections; a powerful immune stimulant; antifungal; analgesic; warming; deodorant; energizing; circulatory stimulant; physically and mentally fortifying; valuable insect repellent

"Winter Thyme" Healthy Home Blend

During cold and flu season, I diffuse this formula — chock-full of antibacterial and antiviral properties — throughout my house, as regularly inhaling it fortifies resistance and general immunity and keeps microbes at bay. The fragrance is fresh, stimulating, and herbaceous, and definitely not medicinal.

ESSENTIAL OILS

40 ♦ thyme (ct. linalool or nonchemotype specific)

35 ♦ rosemary (ct. verbenon; ct. cineole; or nonchemotype specific)

30 ♦ eucalyptus (species *globulus*, *radiata*, or *smithii*)

25 ♦ tea tree

15 ♦ lemon

5 ♦ clove

¼-ounce dark glass bottle with a screw cap or orifice reducer cap

Caution: Do not use in close proximity to children 10 years of age or younger, as it can be too stimulating to the respiratory tract.

TO MAKE THE BLEND: Combine the thyme, rosemary, eucalyptus, tea tree, lemon, and clove essential oils in the bottle. Screw the top on the bottle and shake vigorously for 2 minutes to blend. Label the bottle and set it in a cool, dark location for 24 hours so that the oils can synergize.

Store at room temperature, away from heat and light; use within 2 years. Do not store the bottle with a dropper top, as the strong vapors will degrade the rubber tip. Store only with a screw cap.

TO DIFFUSE THE ESSENTIAL OILS: Shake well before using. Follow the manufacturer's directions for your brand of diffuser or nebulizer.

TO MAKE A SPRAY: Add 30 drops of the blend to a 4-ounce plastic or dark glass spray bottle. Then add ¼ cup of water and ¼ cup of unflavored vodka. Screw the top on the bottle and shake vigorously to blend. Label the bottle and allow the spray to synergize for 1 hour. Store at room temperature, away from heat and light; use within 1 year. Shake well before using. Spray several times per day during cold and flu season. You can also spray the blend on your hands after washing as an added layer of wellness protection; I suggest placing a bottle by the kitchen sink and in each bathroom.

Essential Four Thieves Sniffy Stick

Here's a handy aromatic stick featuring the same antiviral and antibacterial essential oils found in Essential Four Thieves Vinegar (next page). Keep one conveniently stashed in your pocket, purse, gym bag, desk drawer, nightstand, and/or medicine cabinet for a quick sniff during cold and flu season. *Safe for folks 12 years of age and older.*

ESSENTIAL OILS

6 ◆ thyme (ct. linalool or nonchemotype specific)

4 ◆ eucalyptus (species *globulus*, *radiata*, or *smithii*)

4 ◆ lavender

4 ◆ rosemary (ct. verbenon or nonchemotype specific)

2 ◆ clove

2 ◆ lemon

Reusable nasal inhaler tube

TO MAKE THE SNIFFY STICK: Remove the cotton inhaler wick from the inhaler tube. Add the essential oils, drop by drop, directly to the wick. Replace the wick in the tube and tightly cap the bottom with the plug. Place the inhaler tube inside its cover and screw tightly to close; add a tiny label. To recharge, simply add more drops to the wick when the scent weakens.

Store at room temperature; for maximum potency, use within 2 to 3 months.

TO USE: Inhale deeply as needed, up to several times per day. For best results, be sure to exhale through your mouth, not your nose.

Caution: If you suffer from asthma, this formulation may be too stimulating. Avoid completely if you are having an asthma attack.

The Top 11 Essentials

Essential Four Thieves Vinegar

A potent antiviral, antibacterial cold and flu preventive called the "Thieves Formula" has been bandied about by herbalists for centuries. My version of this famous vinegar relies on essential oils instead of herbs. The original formula is said to have been used by thieves during the bubonic plague or "Black Death" of the Middle Ages. Supposedly the thieves who used it while stealing valuables from the dead and dying never got sick.

Use this strongly aromatic topical remedy before, during, and after cold and flu season as a protective agent. If you do succumb, continue using it to ease symptoms and speed recovery. The benefit is derived via inhalation of the herbal properties as well as absorption into your bloodstream through the pores of your skin. *Safe for folks 12 years of age and older. This formula may sting slightly if applied to broken skin. It is intended for topical use only.*

ESSENTIAL OILS

18 ◆ thyme (ct. linalool or non-chemotype specific)

16 ◆ lavender

16 ◆ rosemary (ct. verbenon or nonchemotype specific)

14 ◆ eucalyptus (species *globulus*, *radiata*, or *smithii*)

10 ◆ lemon

6 ◆ clove

BASE

¾ cup apple cider vinegar (preferably organic and unpasteurized)

¼ cup purified water

8-ounce plastic or dark glass spritzer bottle

TO MAKE THE VINEGAR: Combine the thyme, lavender, rosemary, eucalyptus, lemon, and clove essential oils in the bottle, then add the vinegar and water. Screw the top on the bottle and shake vigorously to blend. Label the bottle and allow the spray to synergize for 1 hour.

Store at room temperature, away from heat and light; use within 1 year.

TO USE: Shake well before each use. Spray the formula onto your hands, then rub the liquid onto your throat, the back of your neck, your chest, your ears, and your temples. Do this two or three times daily. Massage the formula into your feet at bedtime and again before getting dressed in the morning. The aromatic medicinal properties will penetrate your nasal passages as well as the thousands of pores in your skin and feet.

I recommend keeping a small spritzer bottle of this formula handy during the height of cold and flu season, so you can use it to sanitize your hands frequently throughout the day.

Bonus uses: Keep a bottle by the sink to spray on hands to eliminate the lingering odor of garlic, onions, or fish; it also acts as an effective hand sanitizer. Applied to fingernails and toenails, it will help get rid of fungus, and it can also be used as a spot treatment for acne blemishes and other minor skin ailments.

Essential Four Thieves Oil

This is another useful application method for the Essential Four Thieves blend, featuring the same antiviral and antibacterial essential oils found in the vinegar (page 104) and the sniffy stick (page 103), but this time in an oil base. Use this strongly aromatic remedy before, during, and after cold and flu season as a protective agent and, if you do succumb, continue using it to ease symptoms and speed recovery. The benefit is derived via inhalation of the herbal properties as well as absorption into your bloodstream through the pores of your skin. *Safe for folks 12 years of age and older. This is an aromatherapeutically concentrated formula, so use only as directed.*

ESSENTIAL OILS

6 ♦ thyme (ct. linalool or nonchemotype specific)

4 ♦ lavender

4 ♦ rosemary (ct. verbenon or nonchemotype specific)

2 ♦ clove

2 ♦ eucalyptus (species *globulus*, *radiata*, or *smithii*)

2 ♦ lemon

BASE

2 tablespoons sunflower, almond, extra-virgin olive, or jojoba oil

1-ounce dark glass bottle with a dropper top

TO MAKE THE OIL: Combine the thyme, lavender, rosemary, clove, eucalyptus, and lemon essential oils in the bottle, then add your base oil of choice. Screw the top on the bottle and shake vigorously for 2 minutes to blend. Label the bottle and set it in a cool, dark location for 24 hours so that the oils can synergize.

Store at room temperature, away from heat and light; use within 1 year (or 2 years if you used jojoba oil).

TO USE: Shake well before each use. Massage a few drops onto your throat, the back of your neck, your chest, your ears, and your temples. Do this two or three times daily. Additionally, massage a few drops into your feet at bedtime and again before getting dressed in the morning. Keep fingers away from eyes, nose, and mouth.

Bonus uses: To treat athlete's foot, massage several drops into both feet (even if only one foot is affected) and between your toes twice daily. To treat fungal fingernails, apply a drop to each nail and massage in thoroughly. For either treatment, repeat application two or three times per day for several months or until the condition abates.

14 Additional Essentials

Bergamot
PAGE 111

Cardamom
PAGE 118

Cedarwood
PAGE 123

Cinnamon
Bark
PAGE 129

Cypress
PAGE 134

Balsam Fir
PAGE 140

Frankin-cense
PAGE 146

Ginger
PAGE 155

Grapefruit
PAGE 161

Heli-chrysum
PAGE 167

Sweet Marjoram
PAGE 173

Myrrh
PAGE 181

Sweet Orange
PAGE 189

Scotch Pine
PAGE 197

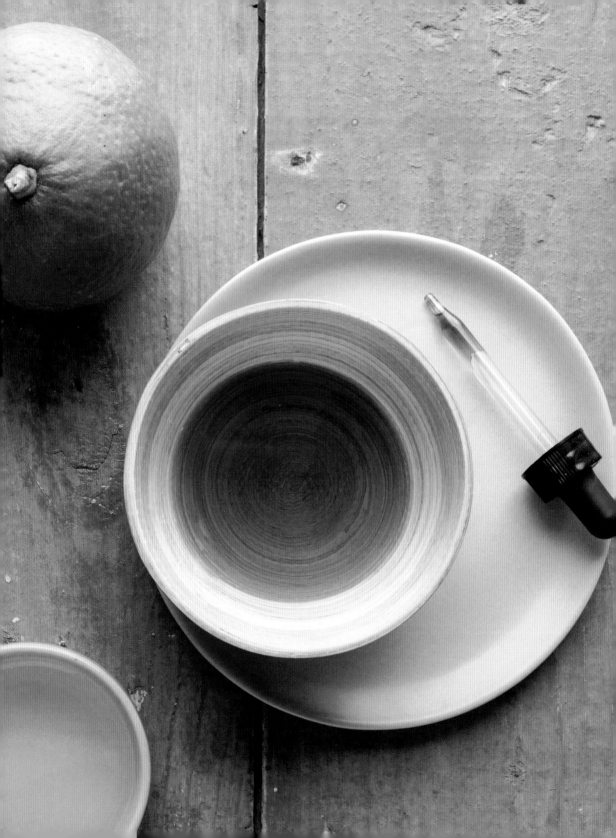

Bergamot

(Citrus bergamia)

Named after the Italian city of Bergamo, where the tree was originally cultivated and the oil first distilled beginning in the eighteenth century, bergamot was used in traditional Italian folk medicine for the reduction of fever (including malaria) and to rid the intestines of parasites. Its seductively floral-citrus aromatic profile is so compelling that it has been used for centuries as a fragrance additive, and it gives Earl Grey tea its distinctive flavor.

Bergamot essential oil's main action is on the nervous system, where its gently refreshing yet deeply relaxing properties help remedy bouts of insomnia and soothe tension headaches, achy or tight muscles, nervous indigestion, hyperactivity, and jitters brought on by anxiety. It's a good oil for stressed-out folks!

It has a particular affinity for relieving skin, scalp, mouth, urinary tract, and respiratory infections. I recommend it for treating stubborn respiratory ailments, slow-to-heal wounds, acne, athlete's foot, and nail fungus. Weeping eczema and psoriasis also respond well to its gentle astringent action, encouraging welcome relief.

A light, clean-smelling, cheerful oil, bergamot is an excellent additive to purifying room sprays, especially when combined with lavender and lemon essential oils, and a hint of peppermint. Makes your home oh-so-fresh and fragrant . . . and inviting, too!

PSYCHOLOGICAL BENEFITS:
Bergamot has refreshing, relaxing, balancing, mood-stabilizing, and elevating effects. Inhaling a few drops on a tissue or a few sniffs directly from the bottle helps relieve depression, anxiety, frustration, and stress-related conditions. It also allays fear and anger and can be of great benefit during times of grief. Bergamot is perfect for the "type A" personality, whose perfectionist, often-critical nature sometimes takes a toll on the skin, digestion, and the nervous system. Women suffering from PMS and the emotional roller-coaster ride that can accompany the transition into menopause will benefit from it as well.

SAFETY DATA: Due to its bergapten content, bergamot essential oil may cause photosensitivity in skin exposed to sunlight and/or tanning beds within 12 hours of use. Otherwise it is nontoxic and relatively nonirritating.

It takes the rind of approximately 100 bergamot oranges to produce 2 ounces of essential oil.

FROM HERB TO OIL

Native to tropical Asia, bergamot is a small, delicate tree with glossy leaves, fragrant white flowers, and small inedible fruits that resemble oranges. Bergamot is extensively cultivated in Calabria in southern Italy (where most of the oil is produced) and also grown commercially on the Ivory Coast. This citrus is not to be confused with the common garden herb bee balm (*Monarda didyma*), also called bergamot.

The light greenish-yellow essential oil, which darkens with age, is produced by cold expression of the peel of the nearly ripe fruit. It has a fresh, fruity-floral citrus aroma with a slightly spicy balsamic undertone.

A *bergapten-free* version of the oil is considered more gentle to the skin, but I feel it lacks vitality compared to the whole oil. Additionally, the intensity of aroma for which bergamot is most famous is notably absent. As with all citrus oils, bergamot has a short shelf life, so use it within 1 year or, if you keep it refrigerated, within 2 years.

ESSENTIAL PROPERTIES

Superior nervous system tonic; emotionally uplifting and antidepressant; gently warming; good antibacterial, antifungal, and antiviral, especially for skin and respiratory ailments; astringent; deodorizing; carminative and digestive aid

Dream Weaver's Relaxing Rub

I chose the essential oils in this formula for their nervine and sedative properties and soft, soothing aromas. When massaged into strategic places on your body, this sleep-enhancing oil blend will lull you into a peaceful state of mind and lead you down the tranquil path to the Land of Nod. *Safe for folks 6 years of age and older.*

ESSENTIAL OILS

25 ◆ lavender

15 ◆ bergamot

15 ◆ grapefruit

15 ◆ sweet orange

10 ◆ Roman chamomile

BASE

1 cup almond, jojoba, or sunflower oil

8-ounce plastic squeeze bottle or dark glass bottle with a pump or screw cap

TO MAKE THE OIL: Combine the lavender, bergamot, grapefruit, orange, and chamomile essential oils in the bottle, then add your base oil of choice. Screw the top on the bottle and shake vigorously for 2 minutes to blend. Label the bottle and set it in a cool, dark location for 24 hours so that the oils can synergize.

Store at room temperature, away from heat and light; use within 1 year (or 2 years if you used jojoba oil).

TO USE: Gently massage a little dab of oil into your chest, back, and temples, around your ears, under your nose, and on your throat. Apply at any time of the day to induce a sense of serenity and relaxation.

Bonus use: This oil blend can be used as a relaxing, blissful bath oil and conditioning lower leg and foot massage oil. It's perfect for easing tense muscles and calming irritable or overexcited children.

14 Additional Essentials

Tranquil Demeanor Balm

Nerves on edge? Anxious? This creamy balm, with its subtle aroma, is guaranteed to take that frazzled feeling down a few notches. The essential oils in this blend infuse your system with incredible soothing effects, leaving you feeling tranquil, yet aware and mentally uplifted. It's perfect for those tension-filled times when you need to relax but don't want to be sedated or overwhelmed with fragrance. *Safe for folks 12 years of age and older. For children aged 6 to 11, reduce the essential oils by half. This is an aromatherapeutically concentrated formula, so use only a pea-size portion as directed.*

ESSENTIAL OILS

16 ◊ bergamot

14 ◊ lavender

8 ◊ geranium

6 ◊ lemon

4 ◊ frankincense CO_2 (if unavailable, use steam-distilled frankincense)

BASE

4 tablespoons refined shea butter*

2-ounce dark glass or plastic jar

*Unrefined shea butter will work, but its stronger fragrance will greatly reduce the already subtle aroma of the essential oils, though not their properties.

TO MAKE THE BALM: Warm the shea butter in a small saucepan over low heat, or in a double boiler, until it is just melted. Remove from the heat and allow to cool a bit for 5 to 10 minutes. Combine the bergamot, lavender, geranium, lemon, and frankincense essential oils in the jar, then slowly pour in the liquefied shea butter. Gently stir the balm to blend. Cap and label the container and set it aside until the balm has thickened, which may take up to 24 hours.

Store at room temperature, away from heat and light; use within 1 year.

TO USE: This is a concentrated formula, so use it judiciously; a pea-size amount or less is truly all you need for the total application. Massage the balm into your temples, under your nose, on your throat, on the nape of your neck, on your chest, or on your pulse points — the wrists, the inside of the elbows, the back of the knees, and just under the earlobes. Rub a dab between your palms, cup your hands over your nose and mouth, and inhale for 10 to 15 seconds. Apply up to three times per day.

Bonus use: The essential oils on their own make a wonderful diffuser blend for the home environment, especially when you're having a stressful day or the kids are ramped up! Combine the essential oils (omitting the shea butter) in a small dark glass bottle (the 5 ml size is perfect) with a screw cap. Shake vigorously to blend, then label and store in a cool, dark spot. Follow the manufacturer's directions for your particular brand of essential oil diffuser or nebulizer, and use the appropriate number of drops.

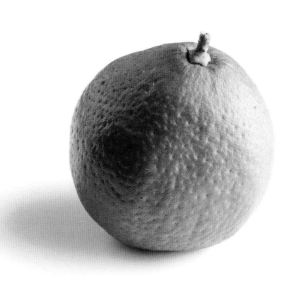

Relaxing Daily Body Wash

Aromatically calming and soothing to the senses, this gentle body wash, with its combination of skin-nurturing ingredients and lovely, subtle scent, produces a creamy lather that leaves skin feeling silky soft and smooth. It's the perfect blend to use in a late-day bath or shower when you want to relax and unwind. *Safe for folks 6 years of age and older.*

ESSENTIAL OILS

8 ◆ bergamot

8 ◆ geranium

8 ◆ sweet orange

6 ◆ lavender

BASE

4 tablespoons unscented liquid castile soap

2 tablespoons plus 2 teaspoons commercially prepared aloe vera juice

1 tablespoon almond, jojoba, or sunflower oil

1 teaspoon vegetable glycerin

4-ounce plastic pump or squeeze bottle

TO MAKE THE WASH: Combine the castile soap, aloe vera juice, your base oil of choice, and vegetable glycerin in a small bowl and mix well. Add the bergamot, geranium, orange, and lavender essential oils. Stir until well blended. Pour into the bottle, screw on the cap, and shake vigorously for approximately 20 seconds. Label the bottle and allow the blend to synergize for 1 hour.

Store in the shower, where the blend will keep for up to 2 months, and then make a fresh batch.

TO USE: Shake well before each use. Apply as a body wash using your hands, a washcloth, or a sponge, working the blend into a light, creamy lather. Rinse.

Bonus use: This formula makes a wonderful shaving product for both men and women.

My Blissful Heart Blend

Here's an uplifting formulation, with light, rosy-citrus-herbaceous notes, for when you are feeling low and blue. It soothes and balances the mind and emotions.

ESSENTIAL OILS

40 ◆ bergamot

40 ◆ geranium

25 ◆ lemon

20 ◆ sweet orange

15 ◆ peppermint

10 ◆ thyme (ct. linalool or nonchemotype specific)

¼-ounce dark glass bottle with a screw cap or orifice reducer cap

Caution: Do not use in small rooms or bedrooms with children under 2 years of age.

TO MAKE THE BLEND: Combine the bergamot, geranium, lemon, orange, peppermint, and thyme essential oils in the bottle. Screw the top on the bottle and shake vigorously for 2 minutes to blend. Label the bottle and set it in a cool, dark location for 24 hours so that the oils can synergize.

Store at room temperature, away from heat and light; use within 2 years. Do not store the bottle with a dropper top, as the strong vapors will degrade the rubber tip. Store only with a screw cap.

TO DIFFUSE THE ESSENTIAL OILS: Shake well before using. Follow the manufacturer's directions for your particular brand of essential oil diffuser or nebulizer and use the appropriate number of drops.

TO MAKE A SPRAY: Add 30 drops of the blend to a 4-ounce plastic or dark glass spray bottle. Then add ¼ cup of water and ¼ cup of unflavored vodka. Screw the top on the bottle and shake vigorously to blend. Label the bottle and allow the spray to synergize for 1 hour. Store at room temperature, away from heat and light; use within 1 year. Shake well before using. Spray throughout the house several times per day, as desired, to help lift your spirits.

14 Additional Essentials

MAKES ¼ OUNCE (7.5 ML)

Cardamom

(Elettaria cardamomum)

For over 3,000 years cardamom has been valued as a domestic spice, especially in India, Europe, Latin America, and Middle Eastern countries. It is employed in both Ayurvedic and traditional Chinese medicine, utilized as a perfumery and incense ingredient, and highly regarded as an aphrodisiac.

The crushed seeds have a smooth, alluring scent and warm, gentle nature that soothes the body, mind, and heart. Cardamom is a relative of ginger and they share several remedial benefits, particularly the ability to warm, tone, and soothe the digestive, muscular, respiratory, and nervous systems.

Cardamom essential oil allays intestinal spasms, eases nervous stomach and nausea, expels gas (it is excellent for colic), improves appetite, and relieves "gastric headaches" initiated by digestive upset. If I'm stressed, my digestive system is the first place to feel it, and I find it simply amazing that these symptoms can be remedied by topical application of diluted cardamom essential oil to the belly and/or feet. Cardamom and peppermint essential oils (my two favorite digestive aids) are *always* with me!

Ayurvedic mouthwash and gargle formulations often include cardamom, as its gentle astringent, antiseptic, analgesic, and deodorizing properties tone and strengthen gum tissue, fight infection, freshen breath, relieve minor throat pain, and help astringe excess mucus from the throat. If you are suffering from hoarseness or laryngitis, cardamom is a good choice to add to a gargle blend. With its wonderfully spicy-sweet flavor, cardamom is also a great additive to lip balm and gloss recipes.

PSYCHOLOGICAL BENEFITS: Cardamom's revitalizing, uplifting aroma is said to open the mind and heart, instilling clarity, joy, warmth, friendliness, and emotional equilibrium; it can help you overcome nervous exhaustion, anxiety, and stress-related conditions. Many find it rather grounding.

SAFETY DATA: Generally nontoxic, nonirritating, and nonsensitizing. Avoid application on or near the face of infants and young children, as it can be too stimulating to the central nervous system and may cause breathing difficulties.

FROM HERB TO OIL

Cardamom is a reed-like perennial herb growing to approximately 12 feet tall, with long, silky blade-shaped leaves. Its lengthy stems bear creamy-yellow flowers with purple tips, followed by oblong reddish-brown pods that appear in clusters at the base of the plant. Cardamom is native to tropical Asia, and the oil is produced principally in India, Sri Lanka, and Guatemala by steam distillation of the dried ripe fruit (seeds).

Most of the world's supply of cardamom is grown for the spice market, with only about 1 percent of the harvest distilled for essential oil. Cardamom essential oil is a colorless to pale yellow liquid with a soft, sweet, warm, spicy scent and woody-citrus undertones.

ESSENTIAL PROPERTIES

Tonic for the digestive system; effective oral antiseptic/breath freshener; revitalizing, uplifting, and balancing to the emotions

Tummy Troubles Oil

This warming oil, with its luscious combination of sweet, spicy, woodsy, and apple-like aromas, leaves your little one feeling cared for and cozy. When massaged into a distressed, achy belly, it delivers relaxing energy plus antispasmodic, anti-inflammatory, and carminative properties — exactly what's needed to soothe and calm the painful spasms of colic and gas. It is an effective aid for mild digestive distress in adults, as well. Using coconut oil in the blend gives the product a comfortingly sweet, warm aroma — I recommend it! *Apply only to the belly, lower legs, and feet. Avoid application on or near the face, as cardamom essential oil can be too stimulating to the central nervous system and may cause breathing difficulties.*

ESSENTIAL OILS

2 ◆ cardamom

2 ◆ Roman chamomile

2 ◆ sweet marjoram

BASE

¼ cup almond, jojoba, sunflower, or unrefined coconut oil

2-ounce dark glass bottle with a dropper top

Bonus uses: This recipe makes a nice foot and lower leg massage oil to calm and soothe cranky toddlers (and adults!), often lulling them into blissful sleep. I love this blend so much that I frequently use it as a "winter warming oil" for the bath or as a massage oil right before bed to help me unwind.

TO MAKE THE OIL: Combine the cardamom, chamomile, and marjoram essential oils in the bottle, then add your base oil of choice. (If you choose to use coconut oil and it is solid or semi-solid, simply set the container in a shallow pan of hot water to liquefy; it melts quickly.) Screw the top on the bottle and shake vigorously for 2 minutes to blend. Label the bottle and set it in a cool, dark location for 24 hours so that the oils can synergize.

Store at room temperature, away from heat and light; use within 1 year (or 2 years if you used jojoba or coconut oil).

TO USE: Shake well before each use. Lay the infant or young child on his or her back, then add a few drops of oil to your hands and rub them together to warm it. Gently massage the oil into the child's belly in a clockwise direction, beginning at the navel and spiraling outward and then down the child's left thigh. This stimulates the colon to release gas and helps quiet spasms. Repeat several times.

"Happy Belly" Foot Rub

All of the essential oils in this formulation are derived from herbs and spices traditionally used to ease symptoms of indigestion, such as abdominal pain, gas, and burping. Designed to be applied directly to the soles of your feet, this fast-acting, pleasantly aromatic foot rub penetrates quickly, delivering benefits to your distressed digestive system. Due to the pain-relieving properties also contained within this blend, it simultaneously helps soothe sore hands and feet while you rub it in. Now that's just good medicine! *Safe for folks 12 years of age and older. For children aged 6 to 11, reduce the essential oils by half.*

ESSENTIAL OILS

- 6 ♦ cardamom
- 4 ♦ ginger
- 2 ♦ sweet marjoram
- 2 ♦ peppermint
- 2 ♦ sweet orange

BASE

- 2 tablespoons almond, jojoba, extra-virgin olive, or sunflower oil

- 1-ounce dark glass bottle with a dropper top

TO MAKE THE FOOT RUB: Combine the cardamom, ginger, marjoram, peppermint, and orange essential oils in the bottle, then add your base oil of choice. Screw the top on the bottle and shake vigorously for 2 minutes to blend. Label the bottle and set it in a cool, dark location for 24 hours so that the oils can synergize.

Store at room temperature, away from heat and light; use within 1 year (or 2 years if you used jojoba oil).

TO USE: Shake well before using. Whenever you're suffering from indigestion, massage a small amount into both feet and put on socks. Repeat several times per day, as needed. Sipping on warm lemon water or peppermint, fennel, or ginger tea is a recommended adjunct to the foot rub.

14 Additional Essentials

MAKES 1 OUNCE (30 ML)

Sweet Spice Protective Lip Gloss

Did you know that thick, glossy castor oil is the primary ingredient in quality commercial lipsticks? Why? Because it conditions the lips, adds shine, and has staying power. Here I've added a smidgen of vegetable glycerin to the mix to enhance sweetness, slip, and hydration. This convenient roll-on gloss, with a flavor and scent that's simply scrumptious, will help keep your lips in tip-top shape . . . plump and kissably soft. *Safe for everyone 6 years of age and older.*

ESSENTIAL OILS

2 ◆ cardamom

2 ◆ sweet orange

1 ◆ ginger

BASE

2 teaspoons castor oil

¼ teaspoon vegetable glycerin

10 ml roller-ball applicator bottle

Caution: Avoid using on sunburned, chapped, raw, or bleeding lips.

TO MAKE THE LIP GLOSS: Combine the cardamom, orange, and ginger essential oils in the bottle, then add the castor oil and vegetable glycerin. Cap and shake vigorously for 2 minutes. Label the bottle and set it in a cool, dark location for 24 hours so that the oils can synergize.

Store at room temperature, away from heat and light; use within 1 year.

TO USE: Shake well before each use. Apply to lips as often as desired.

VIRGINIA
Cedarwood
(Juniperus virginiana)

Virginia cedarwood is actually a type of juniper, not a member of the cedar (*Cedrus*) genus. It is the primary source of most "cedar oil" on the market and most wooden pencils. The familiar, fragrant, red-streaked wood and its oil have been used for thousands of years as an effective insect and vermin repellent.

Native Americans valued the leaves, twigs, bark, and berries for medicine, using a decoction or strong tea, both orally and topically, to treat a variety of ailments, including rheumatism, arthritis, skin rashes, delayed menstruation, venereal warts, gonorrhea, and kidney, urinary, and respiratory infections. The branches were often burned to fumigate and purify the air to ward off infectious disease.

Cedarwood essential oil tones and tightens tissue, gently improving sluggish blood and lymphatic flow, so I like to use it in massage oil formulations (often mixed with cypress and grape-fruit essential oils) for those with a weak venous system (exhibiting varicose and spider veins) and edema. It's also suggested to combat cellulite. For reviving tired, achy legs and relieving the pain of rheumatism — especially when combined with Scotch pine essential oil – it can't be beat!

Cedarwood oil has a wonderfully beneficial effect on the respiratory tract, especially with conditions exhibiting excess mucus, making it quite effective during bouts of bronchitis, colds, flu, phlegm-filled coughs, and other congestive respiratory conditions.

The essential oil's astringent, antifungal, and cleansing properties also greatly benefit conditions of oily skin and hair, cystic acne, seborrhea, dandruff, athlete's foot, and hemorrhoids.

PSYCHOLOGICAL BENEFITS:
Cedarwood has an uplifting yet relaxing effect on the mind and is recommended for those suffering from general debility, mental fatigue, aggression, anxiety, fear, nervous tension, and stress-related disorders. The scent builds emotional fortitude and stabilizes emotions by grounding an individual; it's perfect when you are feeling emotionally drained.

SAFETY DATA: Generally considered nontoxic, but it has the potential to cause skin irritation and sensitization in some. Use in moderation and always diluted. Avoid during pregnancy.

FROM HERB TO OIL

Native to North America, cedarwood is a slow-growing coniferous tree that can attain a rather majestic stature with a height of 110 feet and a trunk diameter of over 5 feet. Essential oil is produced in the United States by steam distillation from the timber waste, shavings, sawdust, and so on. A colorless to yellowish-orange liquid, it has the mild woodsy-sweet, somewhat balsamic fragrance that we associate with cedar chests and freshly sharpened pencils.

ESSENTIAL PROPERTIES

Circulatory stimulant and decongestant; gentle astringent and diuretic; good respiratory antiseptic and mucolytic (loosens mucus); antifungal, warming; deodorant; fortifying and stabilizing for the mind, fighting mental fatigue and emotional exhaustion with a gentle hand; valuable insect repellent

14 Additional Essentials

"Fly Away" Insect Repellent Spray

Oh my, does this repellent smell fabulous — light and woodsy-green, with the zing of lemon. It's a scent that appeals to both kids and adults. Biting bugs, though, will find you less than appetizing and seek tastier flesh! This spray is most effective when insects are mildly to moderately hungry. *Safe for folks 6 years of age and older.*

ESSENTIAL OILS

40 ● cedarwood

20 ● thyme (ct. linalool or nonchemotype specific)

15 ● lemon

BASE

1 cup unflavored vodka

½ teaspoon vegetable glycerin

Rind of 1 lemon, cut into long, thin strips

8-ounce plastic or dark glass spritzer bottle

TO MAKE THE SPRAY: Combine the cedarwood, thyme, and lemon essential oils in the bottle, then add the vodka, glycerin, and lemon rind. Screw the top on the bottle and shake vigorously to blend. Label the bottle and allow the spray to synergize for 1 hour. Leave the rind in the bottle for up to 1 month, then remove it.

Store at room temperature, away from heat and light; use within 1 year.

TO USE: Shake well before each use. Apply liberally to the skin and clothing as needed. You may need to reapply it every 20 to 30 minutes.

Bonus uses: This formula makes a terrific odor-busting underarm and foot deodorant, as well as a gentle yet powerful home insecticide spray. How's that for a multiuse product?

MAKES 8 OUNCES (240 ML)

14 Additional Essentials

Stress-Less Sniffy Stick

Agitated? Irritated? Anxious? Feeling tense and high-strung? Take a few whiffs of this aromatic stick, with its woody-citrus-floral scent — a calmer, more settled you awaits! *Safe for folks 12 years of age and older. For children aged 6 to 11, reduce the essential oils by half.*

ESSENTIAL OILS

8 ◆ cedarwood

4 ◆ bergamot

4 ◆ geranium

4 ◆ lavender

4 ◆ sweet orange

Reusable nasal inhaler tube

TO MAKE THE SNIFFY STICK: Remove the cotton inhaler wick from the inhaler tube. Add the essential oils, drop by drop, directly to the wick. Replace the wick in the tube and tightly cap the bottom with the plug. Place the inhaler tube inside its cover and screw tightly to close; add a tiny label. To recharge, simply add more drops to the wick when the scent weakens.

Store at room temperature; for maximum potency, use within 2 to 3 months.

TO USE: Inhale deeply as needed, up to several times per day. For best results, exhale through your mouth, not your nose.

EO Extra: Cedarwood

To make a disinfecting, deodorizing foot spray for use in my reflexology practice, I often combine 20 drops of fresh, woodsy cedarwood, 10 drops of lemon, and one-quarter cup each of water and 80-proof vodka in a 4-ounce spray bottle. It doubles as a purifying room freshener and underarm deodorant. Clients love it!

Let's Focus! Roll-On Concentration Aid

When you're studying for exams, preparing a presentation for work, feeling artistic, or even meditating, this convenient, pocket-size "focus formula" is just the ticket to help your brain stay in the zone. It combines cognitive-stimulating and balancing essential oils to enhance circulation, aid concentration, and boost memory. Don't let the mild aroma fool you, the blend is quite effective — it's just not overwhelming to the nose. *Safe for folks 12 years of age and older. This is an aromatherapeutically concentrated formula, so use only as directed.*

ESSENTIAL OILS

- 5 ◆ cedarwood
- 4 ◆ rosemary (ct. verbenon or nonchemotype specific)
- 3 ◆ frankincense CO_2 (if unavailable, use steam-distilled frankincense)
- 2 ◆ lemon
- 2 ◆ sweet orange
- 1 ◆ clove

BASE

- 2 teaspoons jojoba or fractionated coconut oil
- 10 ml roller-ball applicator bottle

TO MAKE THE BLEND: Combine the cedarwood, rosemary, frankincense, lemon, orange, and clove essential oils in the bottle, then add your base oil of choice. Cap and shake vigorously for 2 minutes. Label the bottle and set it in a cool, dark location for 24 hours so that the oils can synergize.

Store at room temperature, away from heat and light; use within 2 years.

TO USE: Shake well before each use. Roll a small amount onto your temples, the nape of your neck, behind each ear, and the base of your throat. Gently massage into your skin. Next, roll some onto one palm, rub your palms together to warm the oil, then close your eyes and inhale the vapors from your cupped hands. Breathe slowly and deeply for a few minutes. Avoid contact with the eyes, nose, and mouth. Repeat several times throughout the day, as needed, to help you refocus on the task at hand.

14 Additional Essentials

MAKES 10 ML

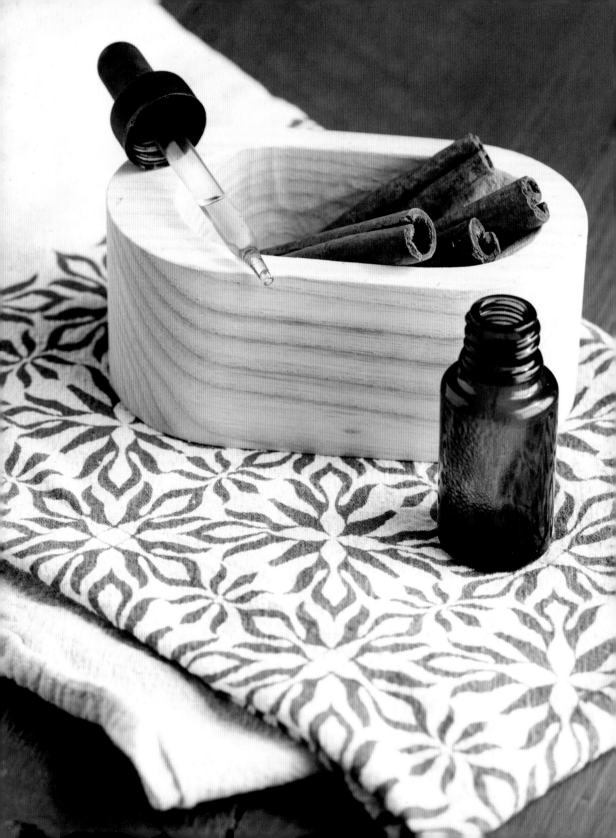

Cinnamon Bark

(Cinnamomum zeylanicum, syn. *C. verum)*

Cinnamon has been an important spice for thousands of years. Owing to its vast number of uses for a variety of disorders, including diarrhea, digestive disorders, menstrual cramps, arthritis, rheumatism, colds, and flu, cinnamon has found a prominent position in traditional medicines, especially in Ayurveda, the traditional East Indian medicinal system.

With its high levels of cinnamaldehyde, the essential oil produced from the bark delivers significant heat. It is generally not recommended for aromatherapeutic home use, unless used in very low dilutions, handled with great care, and given much respect. A little of this one truly goes a long, long way.

Cinnamon is one of the best essential oils for improving circulation, as it really gets things moving. If something is stagnant and stuck or cold and thick — blood, mucus, sluggish digestion, immobile joints, even thoughts — cinnamon helps push it in the right direction.

I don't use cinnamon bark essential oil often except in a few recipes to add flavor to toothpicks, lip glosses, and dentifrices and stimulating, circulatory-enhancing warmth to arthritis, rheumatism, and achy muscle formulations. I also utilize its anti-infectious properties in blends for preventing or reducing cold and flu symptoms.

PSYCHOLOGICAL BENEFITS: The smell of cinnamon bark is like comfort food for the brain. Its inviting scent steadies the nerves, invigorates the senses, eases nervous exhaustion, and allays stress-related debility. It is said to unlock feelings of abundance.

SAFETY DATA: Cinnamon bark essential oil is considered a potent dermal irritant, sensitizer, and mucous membrane irritant. Always use it in moderation and highly diluted. Repeated topical application with minimal dilution can result in extreme dermatitis for some people. Direct inhalation from the bottle or used on its own in a diffuser may result in eye and respiratory irritation. Please use as directed in recipes or in low dilutions of 0.5 percent or less. Do not use if pregnant or breastfeeding. Avoid ingestion of the essential oil if you are taking anticoagulant or diabetic medications, following major surgery, or if you suffer from peptic ulcer, hemophilia, or another bleeding disorder.

FROM HERB TO OIL

Native to tropical Asia, Sri Lanka, Madagascar, the Comoros Islands, South India, Burma, and Indochina, this aromatic evergreen tree, growing to approximately 50 feet, has thick scabrous bark with young shoots speckled greenish-orange. The small white flowers give way to oval bluish-white berries. The essential oil, primarily produced in Sri Lanka and Madagascar, is steam-distilled from the dried inner bark of the young twigs.

Cinnamon bark essential oil is a pale to dark yellow liquid with a sweet, spicy, tenacious aroma. It has a deeper, richer, and sweeter scent than cinnamon leaf essential oil. Its intensity can quickly alter the scent — and heat — if too much is added to a blend of other essential oils. Always use a light hand with cinnamon!

When purchasing cinnamon bark essential oil, be sure that it is sweetly scented, not acidic or harsh, or it will dominate and ruin a blend.

ESSENTIAL PROPERTIES

Hot, powerful circulatory stimulant; a highly effective anti-infectious agent, serving as a broad-spectrum antibacterial, antiviral, and antifungal; good analgesic; energizing; comforting scent for the emotions

14 Additional Essentials

Spiced Chai Breath Spray

This tongue-tingling, lightly sweet breath spray is made with the familiar flavors of spiced chai tea. The essential oils not only neutralize odor-causing bacteria and any unpleasant food flavors lingering in your mouth but also act as digestive aids. I suggest making several bottles of this tasty and useful formula and keeping them on hand at home and at work. *Safe for folks 12 years of age and older.*

ESSENTIAL OILS

- 1 ◢ cardamom
- 1 ◢ cinnamon bark
- 1 ◢ clove
- 1 ◢ ginger
- 1 ◢ sweet orange

ESSENTIAL OILS

- 4 teaspoons purified water
- 1 teaspoon vegetable glycerin
- 1 teaspoon unflavored vodka
- 1-ounce plastic or dark glass spritzer bottle

TO MAKE THE SPRAY: Combine the cardamom, cinnamon, clove, ginger, and orange essential oils in the bottle, then add the water, glycerin, and vodka. Screw the top on the bottle and shake vigorously to blend. Label the bottle and allow the spray to synergize for 1 hour.

Store at room temperature, away from heat and light; use within 1 year.

TO USE: Shake the bottle immediately before each use. Spray once or twice in your mouth to cleanse and freshen your breath.

14 Additional Essentials

Cinna-Mint Glossy Lip Treat

A scent-sational, conditioning lip gloss that tastes lip-smackin' good while freshening your breath, too! Made similarly to Sweet Spice Protective Lip Gloss (page 122), using thick, shiny castor oil as the base and a smidgen of sweet vegetable glycerin, but for this lip treat I added a combination of hot cinnamon and cooling peppermint essential oils. You just gotta try it! *Safe for everyone 6 years of age and older.*

ESSENTIAL OILS

2 ◆ cinnamon bark

2 ◆ peppermint

BASE

2 teaspoons castor oil

¼ teaspoon vegetable glycerin

10 ml roller-ball applicator bottle

Caution: Avoid using on sunburned, chapped, raw, or bleeding lips.

TO MAKE THE LIP GLOSS: Combine the cinnamon and peppermint essential oils in the bottle, then add the castor oil and vegetable glycerin. Cap and shake vigorously for 2 minutes. Label the bottle and set it in a cool, dark location for 24 hours so that the oils can synergize.

Store at room temperature, away from heat and light; use within 1 year.

TO USE: Shake well before each use. Apply to lips as often as desired.

Tasty, Tingly Herbal Toothpicks

Cinnamon-flavored toothpicks, often available for free by the cash register at restaurants, are a super-tasty, convenient way to remove food debris from between your teeth, stimulate your gums, and freshen your breath. I frequently keep a jar of these spicy delights on my kitchen counter. They're incredibly simple to make, and kids (over 12 years of age), not to mention adults, love them!

You'll need a half to a full box (depending on how many you want to make) of quality wooden toothpicks (the round or flat style), a shallow glass jar or custard cup with a lid, and enough cinnamon bark essential oil (or try peppermint, sweet orange, clove, ginger, cardamom, or tea tree) to cover the toothpicks.

Place the toothpicks horizontally in the container, pour in enough essential oil to completely cover them, tighten the lid, and allow them to absorb the essential oil for a couple of days. Remove them from the jar with clean tweezers (not your fingers) and lay them in a single layer on a plate covered with a few sheets of paper towels. Allow them to dry for an hour or two. Store them in an airtight glass jar or tin. The leftover essential oil is perfectly good to use again, so as long as the toothpicks and your hands stayed clean, you can return it to the original bottle.

You can use these toothpicks whenever you want to — just be careful not to rub your eyes or nose after using the toothpick, as any remaining residue will surely irritate mucous membranes. Depending on the flavor, they just might satisfy your sweet tooth, too!

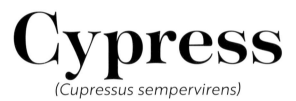

Cypress

(Cupressus sempervirens)

Since ancient times, the cypress tree has been highly valued for its potent astringent, drying, and binding properties, which help moderate excessive loss of bodily fluids, particularly through menstruation, diarrhea, and profuse perspiration; it is also prized for its powerful toning action on the scalp, skin, and venous system.

I use cypress essential oil often, especially in my reflexology and holistic skin care practice. It's beneficial in conditions where there is excessive release of bodily fluids, as in profuse sweating, weeping eczema and psoriasis, cuts or scrapes that won't stop bleeding, and very oily skin or scalp. It stanches, or astringes, the flow of fluids, aiding in normalization and healing. On the flip side, cypress oil is also an excellent herbal diuretic, being of much benefit in conditions of poor circulation in which fluids are retained. Its powerful draining action is recommended for conditions such as cellulitis, cystic and pustular acne, cystic breasts, hemorrhoids, edema, varicose and spider veins, cellulite, lymphedema, and respiratory congestion.

In a gargle, cypress essential oil tones bleeding gums, fights bad breath, relieves the pain and inflammation of a sore throat, and astringes excess mucus in the oral cavity. It's great if you're suffering from hoarseness or laryngitis.

seeming to calm runaway minds. It creates a feeling of security and is recommended for those suffering from nervous tension, restlessness, absent-mindedness, anger, irritability, PMS, stressful menopause, or anxiety. The scent is beneficial for those dealing with the heaviness of grief or emotional crises, as it gently cultivates mental fortitude and stamina, helping people move forward and get on with their lives.

PSYCHOLOGICAL BENEFITS: Cypress is uplifting to the psyche, yet it relaxes, soothes, and grounds the emotions,

SAFETY DATA: Generally considered nontoxic, nonirritating, and nonsensitizing.

One of the folk names for cypress is "tree of death." The Greeks and Romans grew cypress trees on their burial grounds, and the Egyptians used the bug- and rot-resistant wood for making coffins. Legend says that Jesus's cross was constructed from cypress wood.

FROM HERB TO OIL

Widely cultivated as an ornamental, cypress trees are a familiar sight in the landscapes of France, Italy, Spain, Greece, and the western United States. This Mediterranean native is a tall evergreen tree, related to juniper, with slender branches, hard reddish-brown wood, and a statuesque conical shape. It bears small flowers and round brownish-gray cones or nuts. The essential oil is produced via steam distillation of the needles and twigs, primarily in Morocco, Spain, and France. It is a pale yellow to olive-green liquid with a refreshingly smoky, sweet-balsamic-woody odor, reminiscent of pine needles.

ESSENTIAL PROPERTIES

Powerful astringent with primary action on the circulatory system; warming; antibacterial; emotionally balancing and uplifting; calming to the nervous system; effective insect repellent and excellent deodorant

Woodsy Citrus Deodorant Spray

With a light, pleasing aroma, this spray is perfect for men, women, and teens who want to (or must) avoid deodorants with synthetic chemicals. It fights odor-causing bacteria, tones and tightens sweat glands and pores, and leaves you feeling ultra-cool and confident. Keep a small bottle with a few cotton pads handy for when you need to freshen up a bit. It's wonderful as a foot deodorizer, too! *Safe for folks 6 years of age and older.*

ESSENTIAL OILS
16 ● cedarwood

16 ● cypress

16 ● lemon

BASE
1 cup unflavored vodka or commercially prepared witch hazel

½ teaspoon vegetable glycerin

8-ounce plastic or dark glass spritzer bottle

TO MAKE THE SPRAY: Pour the vodka into the bottle. Add the glycerin, then the cedarwood, cypress, and lemon essential oils. Screw the top on the bottle and shake vigorously to blend. Label the bottle and allow the spray to synergize for 1 hour.

Store at room temperature, away from heat and light; use within 1 year.

TO USE: Shake well before each use. Spray onto clean, dry underarms and/or feet, or apply with a cotton pad or cloth and rub in. Let dry before getting dressed. Follow with a natural deodorizing body powder, if desired.

Bonus uses: This formula doubles as an astringent and mild antiseptic liquid cleanser for your hands, face, or entire body, for that matter (avoid the eyes, nose, and mouth). Use for impromptu cleansing when a bath or shower is not convenient. It also makes an effective all-natural mosquito repellent!

Awake and Alert! Sniffy Stick

For times when you need to be wide-eyed and bushy-tailed, here's a stimulating, aromatic inhaler blend with a sharp, woody-fresh scent. This formula will aid in increasing circulation to your brain, delivering a burst of balanced energy. *Safe for folks 12 years of age and older.*

ESSENTIAL OILS

- 8 ◆ cypress

- 6 ◆ rosemary (ct. cineole or nonchemotype specific)

- 4 ◆ eucalyptus (species *globulus*, *radiata*, or *smithii*)

- 4 ◆ peppermint

- 2 ◆ lemon

  Reusable nasal inhaler tube

TO MAKE THE SNIFFY STICK: Remove the cotton inhaler wick from the inhaler tube. Add the essential oils, drop by drop, directly to the wick. Replace the wick in the tube and tightly cap the bottom with the plug. Place the inhaler tube inside its cover and screw tightly to close; add a tiny label. To recharge, simply add more drops to the wick when the scent weakens.

Store at room temperature; for maximum potency, use within 2 to 3 months.

TO USE: Inhale deeply as needed, up to several times per day. For best results, be sure to exhale through your mouth, not your nose.

Bonus use: With antiseptic properties galore, this aromatic stick makes the perfect inhaler to ward off nasty germs during cold and flu season.

Caution: If you suffer from asthma, this formulation may be too stimulating. Avoid completely if you are having an asthma attack.

MAKES 1 STICK

Soothing Hemorrhoid Wipes

The subject of hemorrhoids is not one most people care to discuss, but if you happen to suffer from them, obtaining gentle, soothing relief is uppermost in your mind. In addition to the itching and burning of irritated rectal tissue, swollen hemorrhoids will occasionally discharge blood and mucus, leaving you feeling less than fresh and quite uncomfortable. The ingredients in this formula work together to tighten and astringe tissue, reduce secretions, cool the burn, and calm the itch, while effectively cleansing and deodorizing the anal area. *Safe for folks 6 years of age and older.*

ESSENTIAL OILS

20 ◆ cypress

20 ◆ lavender

8 ◆ geranium

BASE

½ cup commercially prepared aloe vera juice

½ cup commercially prepared witch hazel

1 teaspoon vegetable glycerin

8-ounce plastic or dark glass bottle with a screw top

TO MAKE THE WIPES: Combine the cypress, lavender, and geranium essential oils in the bottle, then add the aloe vera juice, witch hazel, and glycerin. Screw the top on the bottle and shake vigorously to blend. Label the bottle and allow the blend to synergize for 1 hour.

Use within 2 weeks if stored at room temperature, or within 6 months if refrigerated.

TO USE: Shake well before each use. Soak a soft flannel cloth, all-natural and unscented baby wipe, or square cotton cosmetic pad with the wash, and use it to wipe the affected area. Use up to five times per day, but especially before bedtime, in the morning, and after each bowel movement to leave you with a fresh, clean, more comfortable feeling.

Herbal Contact Dermatitis Relief Spray

The term *contact dermatitis* simply means an inflammation of the skin resulting from contact with an irritating or allergenic substance, be it a synthetic chemical, a cosmetic, or a plant such as poison ivy or stinging nettle. Symptoms often include intense itching, a red rash, thickening and inflammation of the skin, blisters that may break open and ooze, scales, and scabs. The rash often has clearly defined boundaries and is generally confined to a specific area of the body.

The ingredients in this mild yet effective formula contain anti-inflammatory, antibacterial, and astringent properties known to cool and soothe irritated, itchy rashes, plus anti-anxiety properties to ease jangled nerves. It smells wonderful, too! *Safe for folks 2 years of age and older.*

ESSENTIAL OILS

10 ◆ cypress

8 ◆ Roman chamomile

6 ◆ lavender

BASE

½ cup commercially prepared aloe vera juice

½ cup commercially prepared witch hazel

½ teaspoon vegetable glycerin

8-ounce plastic or dark glass spritzer bottle

TO MAKE THE SPRAY: Combine the cypress, chamomile, and lavender essential oils in the bottle, then add the aloe vera juice, witch hazel, and glycerin. Screw the top on the bottle and shake vigorously to blend. Label the bottle and allow to synergize for 1 hour.

If you want to keep a small bottle unrefrigerated, perhaps in your purse, briefcase, gym bag, or backpack, it will keep for up to 2 weeks; the spray will keep for up to 6 months if refrigerated.

TO USE: Shake well before using. Cleanse the affected area by spraying with this formula and patting dry with a soft cloth. Then spray once again and allow to air-dry. Use three times daily, or as needed.

Bonus use: This remedy also aids in healing bedsores or skin ulcers, minor burns, hemorrhoids, ingrown hairs, and bug bites and stings.

14 Additional Essentials

MAKES 8 OUNCES (240 ML)

Balsam Fir

(Abies balsamea)

With its clean, alluring fragrance, the honey-like sap of the balsam fir is collected by puncturing the plump blisters that form on the tree's bark. Applied externally, it has been traditionally used to treat burns, sores, cuts, cracked skin, wounds, and chest pain. The tree needles make a bitter, astringent tea that can be used as a wound wash and drunk to treat colds and flu symptoms, coughs, and respiratory infection, and to relieve muscle spasms and general and joint achiness.

This is my absolute favorite medicine tree. I harvest the oleoresin — a rather laborious though enjoyable process — in late spring, when it's plentiful. I blend it into salves to energize my mind, open respiratory channels, relieve headaches, and soften my hands and feet.

Applied topically in formulation blends, clean, tingly-fresh balsam fir essential oil treats and comforts the same symptoms and ailments as the fresh oleoresin and needle tea. It's one of my absolute favorite oils. Inhaling it directly from the bottle or diffusing it in my home lifts mental fog and infuses my brain with a balanced, happy energy like no other oil! Because this oil resonates so deeply with me, I use it in many of my own personal oil blends and salves. It's definitely my "essential oil ally" for health! I truly expect it to work for me, and it does! If your mind thinks you will be healed, half the battle is already won!

PSYCHOLOGICAL BENEFITS: The scent of fir essential oil is often described as opening, elevating, appeasing, relaxing, and grounding. Like walking through an evergreen forest, it opens your respiratory channels and makes you feel incredibly balanced, in harmony with life. It's recommended for those suffering from nervous tension, stress-related conditions, depression, or the winter blues.

SAFETY DATA: Generally nontoxic, nonirritating, and nonsensitizing. Fir essential oil has a rather short shelf life because it oxidizes quickly, so use within 1 year or keep it refrigerated and use within 2 years.

FROM HERB TO OIL

Native to North America, this tall, graceful evergreen grows to 65 feet high, with a tapering trunk, numerous branches, and slender, upright cones. Special vesicles beneath the bark form blisters filled with oleoresin, which is a mixture of essential oil and resin (the so-called balsam), on the trunk and branches. The essential oil is extracted primarily in Canada by steam distillation from the needles and twigs. The essential oil is a colorless liquid with a fresh, soft evergreen odor and a somewhat sweet-fruity-balsamic undertone.

ESSENTIAL PROPERTIES

Ultra-refreshing and uplifting; eases stress conditions; gentle, warming circulatory stimulant; promotes healing of skin irritations and wounds; antiseptic respiratory decongestant and expectorant — loosens mucus, lessens coughing; muscular antispasmodic; remarkable air purifier

Energize and Revitalize Treatment Oil

Feeling tired and achy from everyday stress, overexertion, sitting at your desk all day, running around with the kids, or a lingering bad cold or the flu? Well, here's your remedy! With its beautiful deep orange hue and pleasingly light, herbaceous, uplifting scent, this blend gently boosts your energy and helps reduce inflammation and pain, while nourishing and conditioning your skin at the same time. *Safe for folks 12 years of age and older. This is an aromatherapeutically concentrated formula, so use only as directed.*

ESSENTIAL OILS

16 ♦ balsam fir

10 ♦ lavender

6 ♦ peppermint

4 ♦ lemon

BASE

2 tablespoons calendula-infused oil (page 211)

1 tablespoon comfrey-infused oil (page 212)

1 tablespoon St. John's wort–infused oil (page 213)

2-ounce plastic squeeze bottle or dark glass bottle with a pump or dropper top

TO MAKE THE OIL: Combine the balsam fir, lavender, peppermint, and lemon essential oils in the bottle, then add the calendula, comfrey, and St. John's wort oils. Screw the top on the bottle and shake vigorously for 2 minutes to blend. Label the bottle and set it in a cool, dark location for 24 hours so that the oils can synergize.

Store at room temperature, away from heat and light; use within 1 year.

TO USE: Shake well before using. This formula is designed as a spot-treatment massage oil for areas in need of comforting — the essential oil percentage is too high for it to be used as an all-over massage oil. Once or twice per day, apply wherever you feel achy, such as your lower back, legs, feet, or neck. Warming your skin first by bathing or using a heating pad encourages penetration of the oil.

Bonus use: This oil also speeds healing and brings pain relief to fresh bruises. Apply by the drop two or three times per day until the bruise fades.

"Fog Lifter" Mind Stimulation Drops

Clean, sharp, and invigorating — this is exactly the type of aromatherapy your brain needs when that "pea-soup brain fog" moves in. A few drops of this refreshing formula go a long way toward boosting mental activity and your ability to focus on the task at hand. *Safe for folks 12 years of age and older. This is an aromatherapeutically concentrated formula, so use only by the drop as directed.*

ESSENTIAL OILS

20 ◊ balsam fir

20 ◊ peppermint

20 ◊ rosemary (ct. cineole or nonchemotype specific)

BASE

¼ cup jojoba, almond, extra-virgin olive, or sunflower oil

2-ounce dark glass bottle with a dropper top

TO MAKE THE DROPS: Combine the balsam fir, peppermint, and rosemary essential oils in the bottle, then add your base oil of choice. Screw the top on the bottle and shake vigorously for 2 minutes to blend. Label the bottle and set it in a cool, dark location for 24 hours so that the oils can synergize.

Store at room temperature, away from heat and light; use within 1 year (or 2 years if you used jojoba oil).

TO USE: Shake well before using. Once or twice a day, when you are in need of mental stimulation and clarity of thought, apply a drop of this oil blend to each temple, the nape of your neck, the base of your throat, and behind each ear. Breathe deeply.

Bonus uses: Use these intensely aromatic drops as an aid in healing cuts, scrapes, bug bites, blemishes, infected ingrown hairs, blisters, or any localized minor to moderate skin infection. They are a wonderful addition to your herbal first aid kit! Also, the essential oils on their own (omitting the base oil) make a wonderful diffuser blend. Just follow the manufacturer's directions for your particular brand of essential oil diffuser or nebulizer, and add the appropriate number of drops using equal amounts of each essential oil.

14 Additional Essentials

MAKES 2 OUNCES (60 ML)

A Walk in the Woods Antifatigue Drops

Are you in the throes of a personal energy crisis? Do you find it difficult to get up and get going? Well, move over, coffee! Herbs with invigorating scents and stimulating properties work amazingly well at energizing your body both mentally and physically, sans jitters and the ensuing letdown. There's a reason that the essential oils in this recipe all come from trees. Have you ever taken a walk in an evergreen forest, breathing deeply of the crisp, resinous air, and noticed how refreshed and lively it makes you feel? These essential oils all possess properties that reduce adrenal, mental, and physical fatigue, while providing a feeling of balanced energy. *Safe for use by folks 12 years of age and older. This is an aromatherapeutically concentrated formula, so use only as directed.*

ESSENTIAL OILS

30 ◊ balsam fir

30 ◊ Scotch pine

20 ◊ cedarwood

BASE

½ cup jojoba, almond, extra-virgin olive, or sunflower oil

4-ounce plastic squeeze bottle or dark glass bottle with a pump, dropper top, or screw cap

TO MAKE THE DROPS: Combine the balsam fir, pine, and cedarwood essential oils in the bottle, then add your base oil of choice. Screw the top on the bottle and shake vigorously for 2 minutes to blend. Label the bottle and set it in a cool, dark location for 24 hours so that the oils can synergize.

Store at room temperature, away from heat and light; use within 1 year (or 2 years if you used jojoba oil).

TO USE: Shake well before using. Massage a few drops into the sole of each foot or onto your chest every morning after showering, or anytime during the day when you need a shot of balanced energy. Alternatively, once or twice per day, you can have someone massage a few drops onto your lower back, directly over your kidneys and adrenal glands, to help reduce adrenal stress. Let the oil soak in for 5 to 10 minutes before getting dressed.

MAKES 4 OUNCES (120 ML)

Bonus uses: If you're suffering from a cold or the flu, massage a few drops into your feet and chest to help combat the chills, soothe body aches, and open respiratory passages, encouraging deep, oxygenating breaths. This formula also makes a pain-easing rub for arthritic hands, wrists, elbows, shoulders, and feet.

EO Extra: Balsam Fir

For an antiseptic air-purifying room spray, guaranteed to freshen your home and combat cold and flu "nasties," make this must-try spritzer: Add ¼ cup purified water, ¼ cup vodka, and 10 drops each of balsam fir, lemon, and cypress essential oils to a 4-ounce plastic or dark glass spritzer bottle. Shake well. Spritz throughout the house several times per day.

Frankincense

CO_2

(Boswellia carterii)

Held in high regard since antiquity, frankincense was at one time almost as highly valued as gold. It is recognized as one of the first spices brought back to Europe from the East and was one of the gifts from the three Magi to the infant Jesus. Incredibly rich and aromatic, it has been burned as an incense to appease the gods and to rid the sick of evil spirits; it is still used during Catholic mass to purify both the body and the soul.

Frankincense resin and the essential oil have a long history of medicinal use by many cultures to treat — among other ailments — arthritis, rheumatism, syphilis, leprosy, inflammatory skin conditions, menstrual cramps, muscle aches, digestive and nervous complaints, and respiratory, skin, and urinary tract infections.

The ancient Egyptians prized frankincense as an ingredient in the embalming process and in facial masks, so it should come as no surprise that today, frankincense essential oil is particularly valued for its affinity for the skin. It preserves skin's youth, helps tone and tighten, and balances sebum production; it is perfect for all skin types. I include it in treatment blends for sunburn, scar prevention, eczema, psoriasis, dermatitis, minor injuries, bruises, and dry, cracked, fissured, or chapped skin. I also include it in formulas for aging skin, with an aim to retain its taut youthfulness.

Adding antiseptic frankincense to diffuser blends and vapor rubs helps loosen and drain mucus and relieve coughing. It's also a wonderful additive to oil blends and salves to help relieve tense muscles and achy joints.

PSYCHOLOGICAL BENEFITS: The distinctive aroma of frankincense has a soothing, grounding effect on the nervous system that can both uplift and calm, harmonizing the mind, body, and spirit. It allays nervous tension, anxiety, stress, fear, and anger; provides stability during depressive states and postpartum depression; and serves as a relaxing aid to women suffering from PMS and/or the emotional swings often experienced during the transition to menopause.

Frankincense has been utilized through the ages to enhance spirituality, having the ability to slow and deepen the breath and preserve spiritual energy, resulting in a calmer, more meditative, receptive mind. Frankincense essential oil is appropriate for those feeling overwhelmed by too many responsibilities and their cluttered, chaotic way of life, who long for more time to pursue spiritual and creative pursuits. This ancient oil will assist with reprioritizing your life, helping you focus on those areas that will bring you greater happiness and satisfaction.

For me, frankincense is an intensely rich and aromatically pleasing oil, and I often add a drop or two, combined with a drop of sharp, zesty lemon, to my small candle diffuser at the end of a particularly stressful day — it grounds me, adjusts my attitude, and brings me back to my center in no time flat.

SAFETY DATA: Generally considered nontoxic, nonirritating, and nonsensitizing.

Frankincense essential oil blends beautifully with almost all essential oils, but especially the citruses, as it modifies their fruity sweetness in a most intriguing way.

FROM HERB TO OIL

This small, handsome tree with abundant leaves and whitish-yellow or pale pink flowers exudes a valuable white sap (oleo gum resin) when the bark is incised. The sap hardens into whitish-yellow to yellowish-amber "tears," which are dried and powdered to be distilled into essential oil or used as incense. Native to the Red Sea region, frankincense is harvested primarily in Somalia, Oman, and Ethiopia and distilled mainly in Europe. I prefer the CO_2 extraction over the steam-distilled version — it is richer, smoother, and sweeter. If CO_2 is not available, then you may substitute the steam-distilled essential oil.

The essential oil is a pale yellow or greenish-yellow liquid with an odor that's warm, complex, heavy, pungent, and strongly diffusive, with hints of fresh terpene and an almost green, lemon-like pepperiness, followed by a rich, soft, powdery, sweet balsamic-woody undertone.

ESSENTIAL PROPERTIES

Strong affinity for the skin; rejuvenates and preserves skin tissue; aids in healing wounds and skin irritations; effective antibacterial and anti-inflammatory; respiratory antiseptic; warming; calming and grounding

Resin, Rind & Root "Start Your Day" Spray

Frankincense modifies the sweetness of citrus peels and gingerroot in a most intriguing way. The stimulating scent with mellow overtones starts your day on an energetic yet balanced note. Both cheerful and grounding, this is one of my favorite aromatherapeutic sprays, especially for my home office and reflexology practice room (my clients love it!).

ESSENTIAL OILS

- 8 drops frankincense CO_2 (if unavailable, use steam-distilled frankincense)
- 6 drops sweet orange
- 4 drops bergamot
- 4 drops ginger
- 4 drops grapefruit
- 4 drops lemon

BASE

- 1/4 cup water
- 1/4 cup unflavored vodka
- 4-ounce plastic or dark glass spritzer bottle

TO MAKE THE SPRAY: Pour the water and vodka into the bottle, then add the frankincense, orange, bergamot, ginger, grapefruit, and lemon essential oils. Screw the top on the bottle and shake vigorously to blend. Label the bottle and allow the spray to synergize for 1 hour.

Store at room temperature, away from heat and light; use within 1 year.

TO USE: Shake well before using. When you awaken, spritz throughout the house, or in the areas where you spend the most time in the morning (that might even be your car). Breathe deeply of the pleasing aromatic vapors. Use as desired.

Bonus use: Containing antibacterial and mild antiviral properties, this blend may be spritzed throughout the house to help keep cold and flu "nasties" at bay; you can also spray it on your hands after washing as an added layer of wellness protection.

MAKES 4 OUNCES (120 ML)

Scar Prevention and Treatment Oil

A scar forms as your skin repairs a wound that has penetrated the dermal or second layer of your skin. It's part of the natural healing process. Rosehip seed oil, rich in essential fatty acids, is highly regenerative, and with continued application, it dramatically increases the elasticity of the skin and stimulates the formation of new collagen fibrils, resulting in a smoother, more toned appearance. With a combination of skin-conditioning oils, this blend synergizes to form a superior scar-preventive treatment when applied to new injuries and a scar-fading treatment when applied to existing scars less than 2 years old. *Safe for folks 12 years of age and older. For children ages 6 to 11, reduce the essential oils by half.*

ESSENTIAL OILS

12 ◆ frankincense CO_2 (if unavailable, use steam-distilled frankincense)

10 ◆ lavender

8 ◆ rosemary (ct. verbenon)

BASE

3 tablespoons rosehip seed oil

1 tablespoon sunflower seed oil or wheat germ oil

2-ounce dark glass bottle with a dropper top

TO MAKE THE OIL: Combine the frankincense, lavender, and rosemary essential oils in the bottle, then add the rosehip seed and sunflower seed oils. Screw the top on the bottle and shake vigorously for 2 minutes to blend. Label the bottle and set it in a cool, dark location for 24 hours so that the oils can synergize.

Rosehip seed oil has a short shelf life (as does wheat germ oil). Store the formula in the refrigerator; use within 6 months.

TO USE: Shake well before each use. If possible, immediately after incurring an injury, clean the area thoroughly, pat dry, then massage several drops of this formula into the surrounding skin, making sure to include the borders of the wound. After it closes, massage several drops onto the entire wound twice daily to prevent or at least minimize scarring. Continue this treatment until wound has completely healed.

MAKES 2 OUNCES (60 ML)

For an existing scar that is less than 2 years old, a twice-daily application for at least 6 months can dramatically fade and soften the scar. Consistency with application is key.

Bonus use: This remedy can be applied twice daily, by the drop, to areas of your face and neck where you notice new wrinkles forming as well as to deeper, existing wrinkles to help plump and nourish the underlying tissue. If you are consistent with the application and with proper care of your skin, expect to see noticeable results within 3 months.

Treating Scars

When treating scars with home remedies, keep in mind that everyone's skin is unique and reacts differently to different products. For additional assistance, consult with your local pharmacist about nonprescription topical scar treatments. Scars older than a year or two, raised scars, long surgical scars, burn scars, or those that develop and deepen over time, such as acne and chickenpox scars, can be difficult to treat with home remedies and should be addressed by a dermatologist if they cause discomfort or negatively impact your self-esteem.

Frankincense "Every Purpose" Balm

This is an essential balm for every medicine cabinet! Conveying notes of resin, balsam, and pine needle — a scent that's subtle, warm, and slightly sweet — this balm is infused with anti-inflammatory, antifungal, and antibacterial properties that help soothe and mend cuts, scrapes, dermatitis, eczema, bug bites and stings, bruises, dry or chapped skin, ragged cuticles, and fissured palms or heels. New scars gradually soften and fade with consistent use of this balm, too. *Safe for folks 6 years of age and older. However, for children aged 6 to 10, you must use the verbenon chemotype of rosemary essential oil, as any other type of rosemary may be too stimulating to the central nervous and respiratory systems.*

ESSENTIAL OILS
10 ◆ frankincense CO_2 (if unavailable, use steam-distilled frankincense)

6 ◆ rosemary (ct. verbenon)

4 ◆ Scotch pine

4 ◆ tea tree

BASE
3–4 tablespoons almond, sunflower, or extra-virgin olive oil (use the greater amount for a softer consistency)

1 tablespoon beeswax

2-ounce dark glass or plastic jar

TO MAKE THE BALM: Combine your base oil of choice with the beeswax in a small saucepan over low heat, or in a double boiler, and warm until the beeswax is just melted. Remove from the heat and allow to cool for 5 minutes, stirring a few times. Add the frankincense, rosemary, pine, and tea tree essential oils and stir again to thoroughly blend. Slowly pour the liquid balm into the jar. Cap and label. Set aside for 30 minutes to thicken.

Store at room temperature, away from heat and light; use within 1 year.

TO USE: Apply a small amount of balm to affected areas, up to several times per day.

Wise Woman Skin Mender

Is your skin unhappy, looking out of sorts, and in need of some tender loving care? If so, please give this ever-so-gentle oil a try. With mega-mending power, it soothes, nourishes, and speeds healing for all manner of irritating and painful skin maladies, including cuts and scrapes, insect bites and stings, minor to moderate kitchen burns (apply only after the skin has cooled from the initial burn), eczema and psoriasis, ragged cuticles, diaper rash, dermatitis, sunburn, or dry, cracked, red, or inflamed skin anywhere on the body.

It's the perfect choice for those with delicate and/or super-sensitive skin, and it makes a wonderful nourishing facial oil for environmentally damaged mature skin. *For children under 2 years of age, use only the calendula- and plantain-infused oils.*

ESSENTIAL OILS
- 2 ◆ frankincense CO_2 (if unavailable, use steam-distilled frankincense)

- 2 ◆ lavender

- 1 ◆ Roman chamomile

- 1 ◆ geranium

BASE
- 2 tablespoons calendula-infused oil (page 211)

- 2 tablespoons plantain-infused oil (page 212)

- 1 400 IU vitamin E oil capsule (optional, but it adds skin-nourishing and antioxidant properties)

  2-ounce plastic squeeze bottle or dark glass bottle with a pump or dropper top

TO MAKE THE OIL: Combine the frankincense, lavender, chamomile, and geranium essential oils in the bottle, then add the calendula oil, plantain oil, and vitamin E oil (if desired). Screw the top on the bottle and shake vigorously for 2 minutes to blend. Label the bottle and set it in a cool, dark location for 24 hours so that the oils can synergize.

Store at room temperature, away from heat and light; use within 1 year.

TO USE: Shake well before each use. Apply as needed to areas of skin in need of comfort and healing.

Bonus use: For a bath oil, add 2 teaspoons of this formula to a full tub, swish to disperse, step in, and soak. It can also be used as a pampering after-bath body oil.

14 Additional Essentials

MAKES 2 OUNCES (60 ML)

Sunburn Rescue Spray

Specifically formulated to relieve pain and to rehydrate, rejuvenate, and soothe sunburned skin, this energetically cooling, tissue-mending, aloe-based spray has antiseptic, anti-inflammatory, and mild analgesic properties. It's extremely gentle and suitable even for those with sensitive skin. *Safe for folks 2 years of age and older. However, for children aged 2 to 10, you must use the verbenon chemotype of rosemary essential oil, as any other type of rosemary may be too stimulating to the central nervous and respiratory systems.*

ESSENTIAL OILS

10 ♦ frankincense
     CO_2 (if unavailable,
     use steam-distilled
     frankincense)

10 ♦ lavender

4 ♦ rosemary (ct. verbenon)

BASE

1 cup commercially
   prepared aloe vera juice

8-ounce plastic or dark
glass spritzer bottle

TO MAKE THE SPRAY: Pour the aloe vera juice into the bottle, then add the frankincense, lavender, and rosemary essential oils. Cap the bottle and shake vigorously to blend. Label the bottle, set it in the refrigerator, and allow the blend to synergize for 1 hour.

Store in the refrigerator. Use within 6 months.

TO USE: Shake well before each use. Spray the affected area as soon as possible. You can also apply this blend by pouring it directly over skin or by using it to soak a cold compress. Repeat as needed several times per day, until the skin is completely healed. Follow with your favorite natural lotion or body oil to seal in valuable moisture.

Bonus use: This remedy can also be used to clean, cool, soothe, and speed healing of any type of mild to moderate skin burn, not just sunburn.

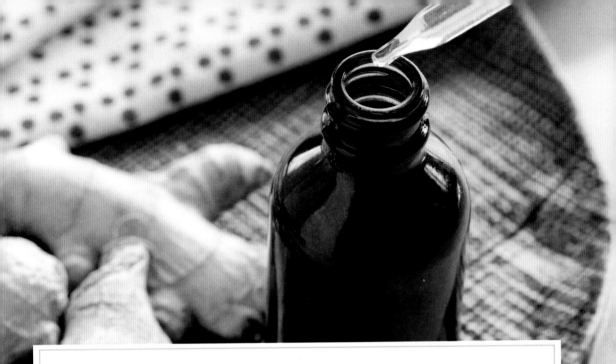

Ginger

(Zingiber officinale)

Delicious and warming, ginger has been used as a domestic spice and remedy for thousands of years in many cultures, especially in the East. With its remarkable healing powers, it remains a staple of both Ayurveda and traditional Chinese medicine and is utilized throughout the world for treating many complaints, including indigestion, flatulence, nausea, toothache, sore throats, sinusitis, malaria, bacterial dysentery, menstrual cramps, muscle spasms, diminished sex drive, and a weak heart.

Gingerroot, whether taken internally in a variety of forms or used as an essential oil, is good medicine for cold, moist conditions where drying warmth is needed, such as excessive "runny" mucus, rheumatism, edema, and diarrhea. It's one of the most widely beneficial warming stimulants. Its main areas of remediation are digestive complaints, including excess gas and nausea; dizziness and motion sickness; fatigue; cold, stiff muscle and joint discomforts; muscle spasms, including spasmodic migraine headaches; sprains, strains, and bruises; poor circulation; and lymphedema. If fluids in the body are stagnant or retained, ginger will help get things moving, and if they are in excess, ginger's gentle astringent action will tone and tighten tissues and reduce flow.

PSYCHOLOGICAL BENEFITS: The comforting scent of ginger energizes and uplifts the psyche, while also being balancing, grounding, and centering. It creates a store of vibrant, radiant energy that promotes feelings of courage, determination, and confidence to help you work through difficulties. Ginger counters mental fatigue, nervous exhaustion, lack of focus, general debility, and lethargy. If you're feeling stagnant or stuck in a rut, or if you frequently get sidetracked from your mission, then ginger is your gal.

SAFETY DATA: Generally nontoxic and nonirritating (except in high concentration); may cause sensitization in some individuals.

FROM HERB TO OIL

From its spreading, tuberous rhizome (root), which is sharply pungent, ginger sends up a green reed-like stalk with narrow spear-shaped leaves and white or yellow flowers. Native to southern Asia, ginger is cultivated all over the tropics. The essential oil is produced in many regions, but especially India, China, Vietnam, Sri Lanka, the Caribbean, and Madagascar, typically by steam distillation of the unpeeled, dried, ground rhizomes. Pale yellow, amber, or greenish in color, it has a warm, fresh, woody-spicy scent that becomes richer, sweeter, and more tenacious as it ages. (There is also a sharper, fruitier, spicier version that's distilled from the fresh root and is exquisite!)

ESSENTIAL PROPERTIES

Analgesic and anti-inflammatory; reduces muscular spasms; strong digestive aid; quells motion sickness; circulatory stimulant; energizing; gentle astringent; respiratory antiseptic and expectorant; warming; appetite stimulant; emotionally uplifting and comforting

"Oral Defense" Tooth Polish

A smoother, milder dentifrice than Sweet Orange–Mint Toothpaste (page 192), this tasty natural tooth polish delivers a winning blend of ingredients containing anti-inflammatory, antibacterial, astringent, alkaline, and mild analgesic properties that help tone and tighten weak and bleeding gums, fight infection, remove plaque, counter acidity, and freshen breath. Due to the inclusion of vegetable glycerin, this formula is quite sweet and extremely thick, so if you prefer your tooth polish not-so-sweet, omit the glycerin and just make tooth powder. For sanitary reasons, make a separate jar for each member of your household. *Safe for folks 6 years of age and older. Gentle enough for those with sensitive teeth and gums.*

ESSENTIAL OILS

6 ⬥ ginger

4 ⬥ peppermint

4 ⬥ sweet orange

2 ⬥ myrrh

BASE

4 tablespoons powdered white kaolin clay

2 tablespoons baking soda

2 tablespoons vegetable glycerin

2-ounce dark glass or plastic container

TO USE: Apply a small amount of paste to your wet toothbrush and brush normally. Do not swallow.

TO MAKE THE TOOTH POLISH: Combine the kaolin clay and baking soda in a small bowl. Mix well, then slowly stir in the vegetable glycerin until the mixture is smooth and creamy, having a texture similar to that of commercial toothpaste. Add the ginger, peppermint, orange, and myrrh essential oils, a drop at a time, stirring constantly, ensuring that they are thoroughly incorporated. Transfer the tooth polish to the container, cap, and label. Allow the finished product to rest for 24 hours so the flavors can mingle and mellow.

Store the container away from heat and sunlight. For best flavor and texture, use within 2 months.

Note: I've made this recipe many times and it still surprises me that pale clay, white baking soda, and clear glycerin turn brown. Despite the earthy appearance of this product, it will not stain teeth; in fact, it brightens them!

14 Additional Essentials

MAKES 2 OUNCES (60 ML)

Clear and Focused Sniffy Stick

Move over, caffeine! Here's a handy inhalation blend of stimulating, circulation-enhancing essential oils that aid in clearing the mind while increasing concentration and focus — without the nervous jitters and ensuing energy letdown that coffee, tea, and soda often deliver. For tasks such as studying or memorization, this aroma stick is especially recommended. *Safe for folks 12 years of age and older.*

ESSENTIAL OILS

- 8 ◆ ginger
- 6 ◆ rosemary (ct. cineole or nonchemotype specific)
- 6 ◆ peppermint
- 2 ◆ lemon

Reusable nasal inhaler tube

TO MAKE THE SNIFFY STICK: Remove the cotton inhaler wick from the inhaler tube. Add the essential oils, drop by drop, directly to the wick. Replace the wick in the tube and tightly cap the bottom with the plug. Place the inhaler tube inside its cover and screw tightly to close; add a tiny label. To recharge, simply add more drops to the wick when the scent weakens.

Store at room temperature; for maximum potency, use within 2 to 3 months.

TO USE: Inhale deeply as needed, up to several times per day. For best results, be sure to exhale through your mouth, not your nose.

Bonus use: With antiseptic properties galore, this aromatic stick makes the perfect inhaler to ward off nasty germs during cold and flu season.

Caution: If you suffer from asthma, this formulation may be too stimulating. Avoid completely if you are having an asthma attack.

Swollen Legs and Feet Spray

Swollen legs, ankles, and feet can be quite uncomfortable, as well as an indication of high blood pressure, rheumatism, constipation, and heart and kidney disorders. Please visit your health-care provider if symptoms recur on a regular basis. If no serious underlying reason exists, then this formula, along with lifestyle and diet modifications, should be most beneficial.

Delivering both warming and cooling energies, this refreshing spray, combined with gentle massage, enhances circulation, encouraging the lymphatic system to drain away excess fluid. *Safe for folks 12 years of age and older.*

ESSENTIAL OILS

16 ♦ ginger

14 ♦ cypress

12 ♦ grapefruit

6 ♦ peppermint

BASE

¼ cup commercially prepared aloe vera juice

¼ cup commercially prepared witch hazel

½ teaspoon vegetable glycerin

4-ounce plastic or dark glass spritzer bottle

Bonus use: The spray may also be used to ease swelling or edema in the arms and hands.

TO MAKE THE SPRAY: Combine the ginger, cypress, grapefruit, and peppermint essential oils in the bottle, then add the aloe vera juice, witch hazel, and glycerin. Screw the top on the bottle and shake vigorously to blend. Label the bottle, set it in the refrigerator, and allow the blend to synergize for 1 hour.

Store in the refrigerator, where it will keep for up to 6 months.

TO USE: Shake well before using. Spray the affected area and massage the blend into the skin using handstrokes and circular motions in the direction toward the heart. This encourages blood flow to return from the affected area to the heart. Use the spray as often as necessary. In hot weather, before massaging the feet and ankles, place a few ice cubes in a plastic bag (or grab a bag of frozen peas) and use them to rub the backs of the knees until they feel quite cold, then rub the centers of the soles of your feet. Alternatively, soak your feet in cold water for a bit.

MAKES 4 OUNCES (120 ML)

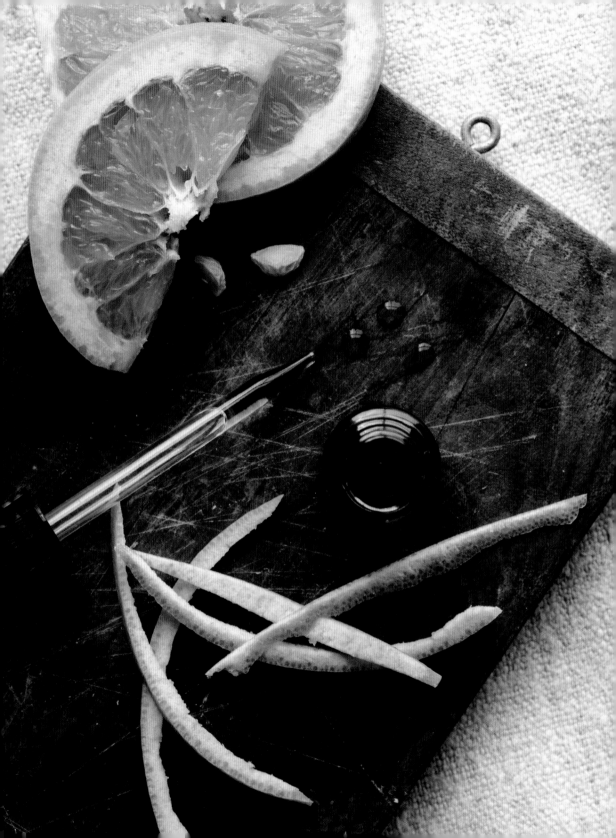

Grapefruit
(Citrus paradisi)

The lusciously sweet-tart, juicy, and pleasingly aromatic grapefruit shares the nutritional qualities of other citrus species, being high in vitamin C, plus delivering ample potassium, folic acid, beta-carotene (red fruits only), and capillary-strengthening flavonoids. It has a stabilizing effect on blood sugar, diminishes the appetite, enhances digestion, acts as a mild diuretic, and offers valuable protection against infectious illnesses. And who can resist the delightfully uplifting scent of the freshly squeezed juice and peel?

Grapefruit essential oil is one of my top picks for massage oils and spritzer blends, often combined with cypress, ginger, and peppermint essential oils, to ease conditions of water retention, fatigued, heavy legs and feet, and general overall achiness. Its astringent action also benefits oily skin and scalp.

Grapefruit offers an amazingly effective and aromatically pleasing cognitive boost that stokes your mental fires, enhancing concentration and mental clarity. I've long adored both the fruit and the oil, as I find the fruit lusciously satisfying and its oil scent-sational. It makes my mind and body smile! Clients love it when my treatment room smells of grapefruit — clean and fresh.

PSYCHOLOGICAL BENEFITS: Grapefruit lifts the spirits, being beneficial during times of depression, overwhelming stress, mental fatigue, and nervous exhaustion. It's especially helpful for the PMS blues. Like other citrus oils, it builds your sense of humor and general feeling of well-being. Grapefruit is an empowering oil, improving your sense of self-worth and confidence.

SAFETY DATA: Nontoxic, nonirritating, and generally nonsensitizing, with only a low risk of photosensitivity

FROM HERB TO OIL

An evergreen that can grow over 33 feet tall, the grapefruit tree has a spreading canopy of glossy leaves, flexible thorns, and sweetly fragrant white flowers. Native to tropical Asia and the West Indies, it is now cultivated primarily in California, Florida, and Texas, as well as Brazil, Mexico, Argentina, and Israel. Much of the essential oil is produced in the United States by cold expression from the outer part of the fresh peel of the ripe fruit. Oil that is distilled from the peel and remains of the fruit after making juice is of inferior quality for aromatherapeutic purposes.

The yellow or yellowish-green liquid has a light, crisp, sweet citrus peel aroma. Grapefruit essential oil oxidizes quickly (as do all citrus oils), so use it within 1 year, or within 2 years if you keep it refrigerated.

ESSENTIAL PROPERTIES

Emotionally uplifting during times of stress; antidepressant; anti-infectious; gently warming; very refreshing and cleansing; detoxifying; appetite suppressant and digestive aid; eases tension and digestive headaches; enhances circulation; astringent and diuretic; deodorizing

Avoiding Grapefruit

Certain medications come with a warning against ingesting grapefruit juice while you are taking them. Why? Because grapefruit juice contains dihydroxy-bergamottin, a chemical compound that interferes with the effectiveness of many medications. Grapefruit essential oil expressed from the peel does not contain this compound, so it is safe to use in aromatherapy for individuals who are avoiding grapefruit juice because of their medication.

"Sunshine-in-a-Bottle" Mist

By their very light, refreshing nature, most citrus oils tend to be rather uplifting to the psyche and particularly good at stimulating a sluggish mind and stagnant circulation, which is why I chose them for the basis of this sparkling, ultra-fresh formula. I added rosemary essential oil for the sharp, energizing, mind-clearing properties that it lends. A few spritzes around my home office with this mist is a sure-fire way to blast out the "mental cobwebs" after an afternoon spent working at my computer!

ESSENTIAL OILS

20 ◆ grapefruit

15 ◆ lemon

15 ◆ sweet orange

10 ◆ rosemary (ct. cineole or nonchemotype specific)

BASE

½ cup unflavored vodka

½ cup purified water

8-ounce plastic or dark glass spritzer bottle

TO MAKE THE MIST: Pour the vodka and water into the bottle, then add the grapefruit, lemon, orange, and rosemary essential oils. Screw the top on the bottle and shake vigorously to blend. Label the bottle and allow the spray to synergize for 1 hour.

Store at room temperature, away from heat and light; use within 1 year.

TO USE: Shake well before using. When in need of mental stimulation, lightly mist your surrounding area and breathe deeply. Use as desired.

Bonus uses: These essential oils contain general antiseptic properties that will help keep your work area and home free of sickness. Spray throughout the house several times per day during cold and flu season. You can also spray the blend on your hands after washing as an added layer of wellness protection; I suggest placing a bottle by the kitchen sink and in each bathroom.

Do not use in small rooms or bedrooms with children under 2 years of age.

14 Additional Essentials

MAKES 8 OUNCES (240 ML)

Happy-Go-Lucky Sniffy Stick

Lighthearted, carefree, uplifted, balanced, euphoric, gently refreshed . . . these are feelings you often experience on a lazy summer's day. This little aromatic stick is formulated to take you there. Just a few sniffs and you're on your way to a better day, emotionally and physically. The scent is citrusy with a hint of rosy-green-resin — most delightful! *Safe for folks 12 years of age and older. For children aged 6 to 11, reduce the essential oils by half.*

ESSENTIAL OILS

8 ◆ grapefruit

4 ◆ bergamot

4 ◆ geranium

4 ◆ lemon

2 ◆ frankincense CO_2 (if unavailable, use steam-distilled frankincense)

2 ◆ peppermint

Reusable nasal inhaler tube

TO MAKE THE SNIFFY STICK: Remove the cotton inhaler wick from the inhaler tube. Add the essential oils, drop by drop, directly to the wick. Replace the wick in the tube and tightly cap the bottom with the plug. Place the inhaler tube inside its cover and screw tightly to close; add a tiny label. To recharge, simply add more drops to the wick when the scent weakens.

Store at room temperature; for maximum potency, use within 2 to 3 months.

TO USE: Inhale deeply, up to several times per day. For best results, be sure to exhale through your mouth, not your nose.

Bonus use: Chock-full of antiseptic properties, this aromatic stick makes the perfect inhaler to ward off nasty germs during cold and flu season.

Potty-pourri Bathroom Spray

The name makes you chuckle, doesn't it? When it comes to eliminating embarrassing bathroom stench, however, this spray is seriously effective. With a sharp, bright scent, plus antibacterial and antiviral properties, this powerful blend can be sprayed directly into the toilet before you use it, creating an aromatic film on the surface of the water, which traps and minimizes offensive odors after your "business" is done. It works wonders if you follow the complete instructions for use below. *Avoid use by children under 10 as the rosemary and eucalyptus essential oils can be too stimulating to the central nervous and respiratory systems.*

ESSENTIAL OILS

24 ◆ grapefruit

20 ◆ lemon

20 ◆ peppermint

16 ◆ rosemary (ct. verbenon or nonchemotype specific)

16 ◆ eucalyptus (species *globulus*)

BASE

½ cup unflavored vodka

½ cup purified water

8-ounce plastic or dark glass spritzer bottle

TO MAKE THE SPRAY: Pour the vodka and water into the bottle, then add the grapefruit, lemon, peppermint, rosemary, and eucalyptus essential oils. Screw the top on the bottle and shake vigorously to blend. Label the bottle and allow the spray to synergize for 1 hour.

Store at room temperature, away from heat and light; use within 1 year.

TO USE: Shake well before using. Spray three or four times directly into the toilet immediately *before* you use it. When you're done, flush, then spray two or three times into the toilet again as it begins to refill with water, followed by two spritzes into the air.

14 Additional Essentials

MAKES 8 OUNCES (240 ML)

Dreamer's Mist

You can't help but be lured into dreamland when you inhale deeply of this delicate mist, with its notes of citrus, lavender, resin, and hints of green forest needle. The essential oils are said to open channels for peaceful dreaming and creative visualization while helping the mind and body relax. I keep a bottle next to my bedside and use it often, as I like to travel in the dream world. *Safe for use by folks 12 years of age or older. For children aged 2 to 11, use only the chemotype verbenon for the rosemary essential oil or simply omit rosemary entirely.*

ESSENTIAL OILS

6 ◆ grapefruit

6 ◆ sweet orange

4 ◆ geranium

4 ◆ ginger

4 ◆ lavender

3 ◆ rosemary (ct. verbenon or nonchemotype specific)

3 ◆ balsam fir

BASE

6 tablespoons purified water

2 tablespoons unflavored vodka

4-ounce plastic or dark glass spritzer bottle

TO MAKE THE SPRAY: Pour the water and vodka into the bottle, then add the grapefruit, orange, geranium, ginger, lavender, rosemary, and balsam fir essential oils. Screw the top on the bottle and shake vigorously to blend. Label the bottle and allow the spray to synergize for 1 hour.

Store at room temperature, away from heat and light; use within 1 year.

TO USE: Shake well before using. Immediately before snuggling under the covers, lightly mist your bedroom, linens, and pillow. Breathe deeply . . . sweet dreams.

Bonus use: This spray works wonderfully well as an aid to calm young children who tend to get irritable just before bedtime. Simply spritz their bedroom on a nightly basis, and they'll soon begin to associate this scent with end-of-the-day relaxation time.

Helichrysum

(Helichrysum italicum, syn. *H. angustifolium)*

The brightly colored, daisylike flowers of this strongly aromatic, shrubby herb can be kept for years in a dried arrangement; in fact, helichrysum is also known as immortelle or everlasting. The name *helichrysum* is derived from the Greek *helios* (sun) and *chrysos* (gold). Usually taken in the form of a decoction or infusion, helichrysum has long been valued for its astounding number of medicinal properties, especially in Mediterranean countries, where it has been used as a remedy for respiratory complaints, liver ailments, skin conditions, headaches, inflammatory conditions such as rheumatism, and muscular aches, sprains, and strains. African cultures prized the plant as a wound healer and burned the fragrant leaves as ceremonial incense.

Helichrysum essential oil is relatively new to the market, but demand for it is high, given its undisputed ability to help heal damaged skin tissue. Extremely gentle but highly efficacious, it is a powerful wound healer, a potent antiaging agent, and a superb anti-inflammatory. I especially like it for its ability to ease arthritic pain, sciatica, sprains, strains, and muscle spasms, including menstrual cramps. It is wonderful for soothing achy hands and feet, too. Like lavender, helichrysum essential oil is a complete medicine chest in a bottle!

PSYCHOLOGICAL BENEFITS: Helichrysum is nurturing, calming, gently uplifting, and harmonizing, which is helpful when you're dealing with issues of depression, apprehension, phobias, stress, lethargy, mental unrest/exhaustion, shock, and irritability. Thought to open the heart, it provides warmth and grounding to those dealing with emotional coldness and fear. It also helps untangle emotional knots and resolve past trauma. Helichrysum has a soothing yet strengthening action; it instills courage and confidence and helps sweeten the temperament.

SAFETY DATA: Generally nontoxic, non-irritating, and nonsensitizing.

Called "poor man's curry" or the "curry plant," helichrysum features golden flowers that have been used in cooking as a substitute for expensive Asian curry spice.

FROM HERB TO OIL

Helichrysum is native to the Mediterranean region and North Africa, and its essential oil is mainly produced in Italy, Spain, France, Croatia, Corsica, Hungary, and Bulgaria. It takes approximately 1 ton of hand-harvested helichrysum flowering tops to produce just over 2 pounds of essential oil by steam distillation. Thank goodness a little goes a long way! The yellow to slightly reddish oil has a powerful, earthy, honey-like scent with a gently spicy undertone.

ESSENTIAL PROPERTIES

Powerful skin cell regenerative, excellent for treating wounds, burns, and skin irritations and pampering environmentally damaged, sensitive, or mature skin; antibacterial; superb anti-inflammatory and pain reliever; gently warming; soothes emotions and strengthens resistance, especially in times of heavy stress

Herbal Comfort: Gout Pain Relief Drops

Gout develops from deposits of monosodium urate crystals in the joints that accumulate due to an abnormally high level of uric acid (hyperuricemia) in the blood. Flare-ups, which can occur without warning, are characterized by extremely painful joint inflammation along with tight, shiny red or purplish skin. The disorder most often affects the joint at the base of the big toe but also commonly the instep, ankle, knee, wrist, fingers, and elbow.

This combination of comforting herbal extracts has a warm, slightly medicinal aroma and a rich amber hue. It boasts potent anti-inflammatory, analgesic, anti-rheumatic, antispasmodic, antibacterial, antiviral, and vulnerary properties. This is effective plant medicine with a gentle hand! *Safe for folks 6 years of age or older.*

ESSENTIAL OILS

5 ◆ helichrysum

4 ◆ lavender

3 ◆ German chamomile

BASE

1 tablespoon comfrey-infused oil (page 212)

1 tablespoon St. John's wort–infused oil (page 213)

1-ounce dark glass bottle with a dropper top

TO MAKE THE DROPS: Combine the helichrysum, lavender, and chamomile essential oils in the bottle, then add the comfrey and St. John's wort oils. Screw the top on the bottle and shake vigorously for 2 minutes to blend. Label the bottle and set it in a cool, dark location for 24 hours so that the oils can synergize.

Store at room temperature, away from heat and light; use within 1 year.

TO USE: Shake well before use. Massage a few drops of the oil into areas affected by gout pain, stiffness, and inflammation. Apply up to three times per day.

Bonus uses: This "herbal-comfort-in-a-bottle" can help relieve the pain of arthritis (especially in the small joints of the fingers, wrists, and feet), backache, muscle stiffness and strains, bruised skin, inflamed bunions, tendonitis, and bursitis. Additionally, a few drops applied to cuts and scrapes helps keep infection at bay while promoting skin tissue regeneration. *Do not apply to open wounds.*

14 Additional Essentials

MAKES 1 OUNCE (30 ML)

Essential Sports Rub

This effective oil blend contains powerful anti-inflammatory, antispasmodic, and analgesic properties and has a subtly sweet herby aroma. It is designed to improve muscular circulation during the warm-up process or to deliver relief from overexertion after any vigorous or prolonged physical activity. It leaves muscles feeling fabulous! *Safe for folks 12 years of age and older. For children ages 6 to 11, omit the rosemary essential oil.*

ESSENTIAL OILS

8 ◆ helichrysum

6 ◆ lavender

6 ◆ rosemary (ct. cineole; or nonchemotype specific)

4 ◆ ginger

2 ◆ sweet orange

BASE

3 tablespoons comfrey-infused oil (page 212)

3 tablespoons St. John's wort–infused oil (page 213)

2 tablespoons calendula-infused oil (page 211)

4-ounce plastic squeeze bottle or dark glass bottle with a pump, screw cap, or dropper top

TO MAKE THE RUB: Combine the helichrysum, lavender, rosemary, ginger, and orange essential oils in the bottle, then add the comfrey, St. John's wort, and calendula oils. Screw the top on the bottle and shake vigorously for 2 minutes to blend. Label the bottle and set it in a cool, dark location for 24 hours so that the oils can synergize.

Store at room temperature, away from heat and light; use within 1 year.

TO USE: Shake well before each use. If possible, have a friend or partner massage this blend into your muscles, paying particular attention to any painful or tense areas, before and/or after activity. Applying it to skin that is prewarmed from a bath, shower, or heating pad encourages the oil to penetrate deeply, but it is not necessary.

Bonus uses: This blend also delivers soothing pain relief to sprains, arthritic joints, and newly bruised tissue. It effectively relaxes and comforts muscle spasms in the arms, hands, legs, and feet, too. Apply to affected areas three or four times per day.

Rapid Pain Relief Remedy

Because helichrysum essential oil is so mild, it can be applied "neat" or undiluted when immediate relief is needed to minimize pain after an injury. A good way to enhance the effect of the essential oil in the treatment of a bruise, sprain, or general muscular trauma is to apply it in combination with comfrey-infused oil (page 212). Add 12 drops of helichrysum to 1 ounce (2 tablespoons) of comfrey oil. Gently massage into the affected area three or four times per day. For children ages 6 to 11, reduce the essential oil amount by half.

Bunion "Pain-Ease" Gel

A bunion is the result of chronic inflammation and thickening of the synovial bursa of the big toe joint, usually resulting in enlargement of the joint and lateral displacement of the toe. A bunionette occurs at the base of the little toe. Bunions tend to be hereditary, though regularly wearing ill-fitting shoes with a tight toe box and/or high heels can encourage them to form. For long-term health, toes need wiggle room, not constriction, and a low heel. If painful bunions are the bane of your existence, try this cooling, soothing, penetrating gel that quickly gets to work at relieving the inflammation, skin irritation, and throbbing pain associated with this common foot problem. *Safe for folks 6 years of age and older.*

ESSENTIAL OILS

8 ◆ helichrysum

6 ◆ lavender

6 ◆ peppermint

4 ◆ sweet orange

BASE

½ teaspoon unflavored vodka

¼ cup commercially prepared aloe vera gel

2-ounce plastic or dark glass jar

TO MAKE THE GEL: Combine the vodka with the helichrysum, lavender, peppermint, and orange essential oils in a small glass or stainless steel bowl; a custard cup works well. Mix thoroughly, then add the aloe vera gel and stir vigorously to blend. Pour the gel into the jar, cap, and label. Allow product to synergize in the refrigerator for 24 hours prior to use.

Store in the refrigerator, where it will keep for up to 6 months.

TO USE: Gently stir before each use, as the essential oils may separate from the aloe vera. Spoon ½ teaspoon of gel into your hand and gently massage into your achy bunion for several minutes. Repeat as needed. Massage any remaining gel into the rest of your foot.

Bonus uses: This aromatherapeutic gel also eases the pain of arthritis (especially in the small joints of the fingers, wrists, and feet), backache, muscle stiffness and strains, bruised skin, tendonitis, and bursitis. Additionally, a small amount applied to cuts and scrapes helps keep infection at bay while promoting skin tissue regeneration.

Marjoram

(Origanum majorana)

Strongly aromatic sweet marjoram, a close relative of oregano, is a traditional culinary herb and folk remedy that was especially favored by the ancient Greeks, Romans, and Egyptians, who utilized in their food, cosmetics, fragrances, and medicines. Introduced into Europe in the Middle Ages, sweet marjoram became a favorite ingredient in bathwaters and body splashes. It was also a prized "strewing herb," placed on the earthen floors of homes to subdue disagreeable odors.

An incredibly versatile herb, having seen use as a tea, decoction, compress, and culinary spice, sweet marjoram has long been recognized as valuable medicine for myriad complaints, including digestive upsets, intestinal cramps, menstrual problems, nervous disorders, respiratory infections, fungal conditions, muscular and rheumatic pain, sprains, stiff joints, bruises, anxiety, and insomnia.

The essential oil is a convenient way to employ the many benefits of sweet marjoram, and it's one of my preferred oils for addressing general arthritic pain, rheumatism, gout, sore or stiff muscles, muscle spasms, menstrual cramps, and migraine headaches with neck tension. Its deeply soothing, warming action brings almost instant relief to all muscle and joint conditions.

As with most oils extracted from culinary herbs, sweet marjoram essential oil is effective for digestive problems, as well as irritable bowel syndrome, intestinal cramps, and infantile colic. When using it in a massage oil blend for anything to do with the digestive system, remember to massage the belly in a clockwise direction, beginning at the navel and spiraling outward, ending at the top of the left thigh, to encourage the digestive process to move in the normal direction.

Being a very effective relaxant, sweet marjoram is an excellent oil to use if you have trouble winding down after getting into bed or if you suffer from insomnia. Place a few drops in your bedroom diffuser and turn it on 15 to 30 minutes before retiring. The soothing fragrance will lull you into restful sleep before you know it.

A good substitute for sweet marjoram essential oil, especially with regard to treating digestive upsets and muscular and joint pain, is Roman chamomile. They share many of the same properties, and both are gentle enough for use with infants.

PSYCHOLOGICAL BENEFITS: Marjoram essential oil is quite tranquilizing to the central nervous system and positively wonderful for easing nervous exhaustion, anxiety, irritability, restlessness, agitation, a racing mind, and other stress-related conditions, including premenstrual and menopausal tensions. It promotes a sense of peace, consoles a grief-stricken heart, and relieves heartache, feelings of rejection, and loneliness.

SAFETY DATA: Generally nontoxic, nonsensitizing, and nonirritating, with possible dermal sensitization in some individuals. Avoid in cases of low blood pressure. Excessive use may significantly lower libido, cause drowsiness or extreme lethargy, or have a deadening or stupefying effect on the mind.

The ancient Greeks called sweet marjoram *orosganos*, meaning "joy of the mountain." As a token of good fortune and to symbolize happiness, honor, and love, newlyweds were crowned with garlands made from the herb.

FROM HERB TO OIL

Also known as knotted marjoram, sweet marjoram is a bushy perennial (cultivated as an annual in colder climates) growing to 24 inches tall with a hairy stem; small, oval, dark green leaves; and small, tightly clustered, pale or dark pinkish-purple flowers, or "knots." Native to the Mediterranean region, Egypt, and North Africa, the herb is cultivated in Egypt, France, Germany, Hungary, Tunisia, Spain, Portugal, and more recently the United States.

The essential oil, which is steam-distilled from freshly dried leaves and flowers, is primarily produced in France, Spain, and Egypt. It is a pale straw or yellow-amber liquid with a persistent warm, pungent, woody-sweet, softly spicy-camphorous aroma.

ESSENTIAL PROPERTIES

Powerful, warming muscle relaxant and antispasmodic; analgesic; deeply tranquilizing to the central nervous system and beneficial for insomnia and stress-related conditions; exceptional sedative; potent digestive agent; strong respiratory antiseptic, countering many infections resulting from a bad cold or flu

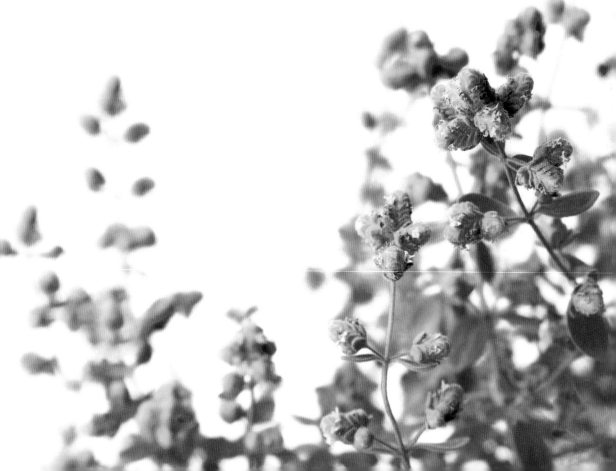

Migraine Melt-Away Blend

Migraine headaches are downright torturous! They have many triggers, from stress, hormonal flare-ups, and food allergies to high altitudes, barometric pressure changes, and bright sunlight, and they are often accompanied by nausea and sensitivity to light and sound. Ugh — the sooner you can find relief, the better!

This formula combines essential oils with analgesic, anti-inflammatory, and antispasmodic properties to deliver powerful, effective pain relief with a gentle, relaxing hand. The scent is rather strong but not overwhelming — aromatherapy at its finest, indeed! If your migraines persist, please see your health-care provider. *Safe for folks 12 years of age and older. This is an aromatherapeutically concentrated formula, so use only as directed.*

ESSENTIAL OILS

35 ◆ sweet marjoram

35 ◆ peppermint

30 ◆ rosemary (ct. cineole or nonchemotype specific)

25 ◆ eucalyptus (species *globulus*)

25 ◆ lavender

¼-ounce dark glass bottle with a screw cap or orifice reducer cap

TO MAKE THE BLEND: Combine the marjoram, peppermint, rosemary, eucalyptus, and lavender essential oils in the bottle. Screw the top on the bottle and shake vigorously for 2 minutes to blend. Label the bottle and set it in a cool, dark location for 24 hours so that the oils can synergize.

Store at room temperature, away from heat and light; use within 2 years. Do not store the bottle with a dropper top, as the strong vapors will degrade the rubber tip. Store only with a screw cap.

TO USE IN A NASAL INHALER TUBE: Remove the cotton inhaler wick from the tube. From your stock bottle, add 24 drops directly to the wick and allow it to absorb the entire amount. Insert the wick inside the inhaler tube and tightly cap the bottom of the inhaler with the plug. Place the inhaler tube inside its cover and screw tightly to close; add a tiny label.

Inhale as needed to bring relief. For best results, exhale through your mouth, not your nose. Depending on how often you open the stick, the medicinal properties will wane and the scent weaken. If your stick is easy to reopen, simply add more drops to the wick to recharge and reuse.

TO USE IN A 10 ML ROLL-ON APPLICATOR BOTTLE: Add 16 drops of the blend to the bottle, then add approximately 2 teaspoons of jojoba or fractionated coconut oil. Cap and shake vigorously for 2 minutes. Label the bottle and set it in a cool, dark location for 24 hours so that the oils can synergize.

To apply, roll a little onto each temple, the base of the neck, and the forehead region. Massage in well. Next, roll some onto one palm, rub your palms together to warm the oil, then close your eyes and inhale the vapors from your cupped hands. Breathe slowly and deeply for a few minutes. Avoid direct contact with the eyes, nose, and mouth. Repeat several times throughout the day, as needed, until your migraine melts away.

Release-Your-Tensions Massage Oil

This blend is an ideal general massage oil that comforts, warms, and relaxes tight, tense muscles and joints anywhere on the body, while calming excess stress and anxiety, leaving you feeling balanced and mellow. It is perfect for an end-of-the-day massage. *Safe for folks 12 years of age and older.*

ESSENTIAL OILS

10 ♦ sweet marjoram

8 ♦ geranium

8 ♦ lavender

6 ♦ bergamot

BASE

½ cup jojoba, almond, sunflower, or extra-virgin olive oil

4-ounce plastic squeeze bottle or dark glass bottle with a pump, screw cap, or dropper top

TO MAKE THE OIL: Combine the marjoram, geranium, lavender, and bergamot essential oils in the bottle, then add your base oil of choice. Screw the top on the bottle and shake vigorously for 2 minutes to blend. Label the bottle and set it in a cool, dark location for 24 hours so that the oils can synergize.

Store at room temperature, away from heat and light; use within 1 year (or 2 years if you used jojoba oil).

TO USE: Shake well before each use. Have a friend or partner massage this soothing remedy into your back, neck, arms, legs, or anywhere your muscles and/or joints are sore and achy. Using it on skin that is prewarmed from a bath, shower, or heating pad encourages penetration of the oil.

Menstrual Cramp Relief Rub

This comforting, aromatic blend of herbal oils with analgesic, nervine, antispasmodic, and anti-inflammatory properties will help ease cramping and relax tense muscles when massaged into the abdomen and lower back. Additionally, the vapors will help relieve the emotional anxiety and nervous tension that often accompany premenstrual syndrome. Though I've included only a small amount of marjoram essential oil, its powerful sedative quality enhances the overall effectiveness of this formula. *Safe for folks 12 years of age and older.*

ESSENTIAL OILS
- 8 ◆ lavender
- 6 ◆ Roman chamomile
- 5 ◆ ginger
- 5 ◆ sweet marjoram

BASE
- 3 tablespoons St. John's wort–infused oil (page 213)
- 1 tablespoon castor oil
- 2-ounce dark glass bottle with a dropper top

TO MAKE THE RUB: Combine the lavender, chamomile, ginger, and marjoram essential oils in the bottle, then add the St. John's wort and castor oils. Screw the top on the bottle and shake vigorously for 2 minutes to blend. Label the bottle and set it in a cool, dark location for 24 hours so that the oils can synergize.

Store at room temperature, away from heat and light; use within 1 year.

TO USE: Shake well before use. Massage ½ to 1 teaspoon of this blend into your lower abdomen and lower back. Cover these areas with a thin, soft cloth, such as flannel, or don an old, long T-shirt, and place a hot water bottle or heating pad on your abdomen. Lie down in a comfortable position for 30 minutes or so, until the pain subsides or at least becomes less intense. Repeat twice daily.

Bonus use: If you suffer from occasional muscle cramps in the arms, hands, legs, or feet, this formula will deliver soothing relief, helping to relax spasms and tension. Simply apply a small amount to the affected muscles and massage it in gently.

MAKES 2 OUNCES (60 ML)

14 Additional Essentials

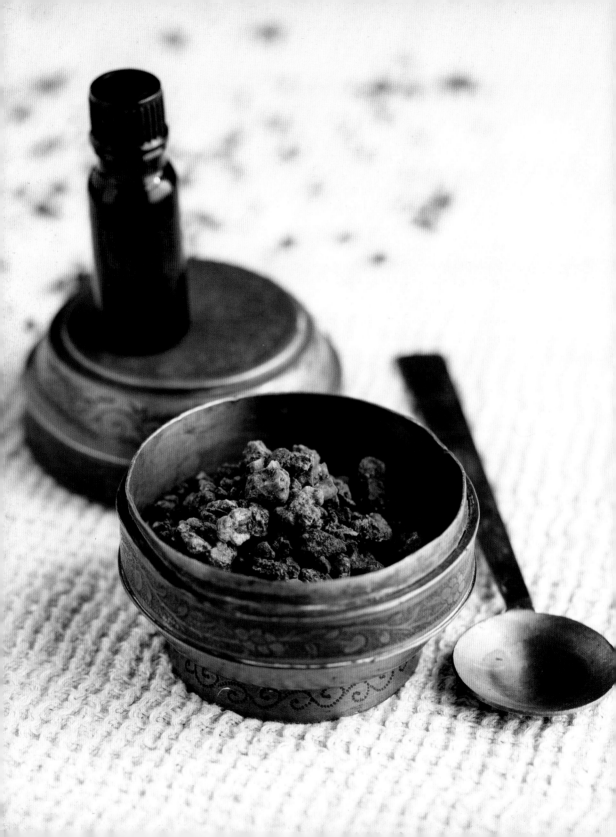

Myrrh

(Commiphora myrrha)

Myrrh's rich, aromatic, precious resin was probably more widely used in ancient times — especially throughout the Middle East — than any other aromatic for incense, perfumes, and medicine. It was particularly prized for its ability to heal infections of the respiratory tract, mouth, and skin and as a digestive stimulant. Myrrh was also one of the three gifts said to have been brought by the three wise men to the baby Jesus to support a state of grace and preserve divine essence.

Myrrh essential oil is valued for many of the same uses as the resin. Known for its rejuvenating and revitalizing effects on the skin, it is often used in antiaging products to delay wrinkling and improve the skin's texture and tone. I swear by myrrh essential oil's "youthifying" effects and always add a few drops to facial oils and creams. It also successfully promotes the healing of all manner of wounds, inflamed skin conditions (such as weeping eczema and psoriasis, hemorrhoids, and acne), and environmentally damaged, dry, chapped, cracked skin.

Myrrh essential oil has a superb reputation as a remedy for inflammatory and infectious conditions of the mouth and throat (bleeding gums, gingivitis, ulcers, bad breath, pyorrhea, receding gums, thrush, general sore throat, laryngitis, and tonsillitis). It's also a strong respiratory antiseptic with drying and purifying properties that help kill infection and loosen and expectorate mucus during cases of bronchitis, sinusitis, asthma, coughs, and colds.

PSYCHOLOGICAL BENEFITS: The centering, grounding scent of myrrh is beneficial in cases of apathy, emotional coldness, weakness, and lack of motivation. It cools heated emotions and calms states of fear, panic, and hysteria. It also fortifies and revitalizes the spirit, building confidence in those who are afraid to speak up about their feelings. It promotes spiritual awareness and is recommended for meditation and prayer; it can also be used to ease the anguish of grief.

SAFETY DATA: Generally nonirritating and nonsensitizing. Avoid during pregnancy and while breastfeeding.

The name *myrrh* derives from the Arabic *murr*, meaning "bitter."

FROM HERB TO OIL

The scrubby, thorny myrrh tree has knotted branches, small three-part leaves, and white flowers. When pierced or incised, the trunk and larger limbs yield a pale yellow liquid that hardens into the reddish-brown drops known as myrrh or myrrh gum resin. These are dried to be distilled into essential oil or used as incense. The tree is native to the Middle East, northeast Africa, and southwest Asia, though its growing range has been extended by cultivation. The essential oil is primarily distilled in Somalia, Ethiopia, and Sudan.

Myrrh essential oil is produced by steam distillation of the crude gum resin. A lovely, sweeter CO_2 is also produced in lesser quantity, as is a resinoid and resin absolute. It is an oily, pale yellow to amber liquid with a rather unique odor: warm, sweet-balsamic, slightly spicy-medicinal, smoky-musty.

ESSENTIAL INFORMATION

Tones and tightens skin tissue; highly antibacterial, astringent, and anti-inflammatory; best remedy for mouth, gum, and throat irritations and infections; powerful respiratory antiseptic and expectorant; stimulating; warming; strengthens and fortifies the emotions; grounding and centering to the mind

Divine Essence

Feeling frazzled, frustrated, flighty, anxious, tense, and fatigued as a result of being pulled in too many directions? Need of a sense of integration? At times when all around you seems to be spinning out of control, diffuse this divine blend, a magical pairing of two precious "spiritual resins" — myrrh and frankincense — into your environment and experience a slowing and deepening of breath, while you become more centered, grounded, and relaxed, but still aware. This formula came to me in a dream at a time when I really needed it. It won't solve your problems, but it might offer a few moments of clarity. *Do not use in small rooms or bedrooms with children under 2 years of age.*

ESSENTIAL OILS

50 ♦ myrrh

40 ♦ frankincense CO_2 (if unavailable, use steam-distilled frankincense)

30 ♦ geranium

30 ♦ lemon

¼-ounce dark glass bottle with a screw cap or orifice reducer cap

TO MAKE THE BLEND: Combine the myrrh, frankincense, geranium, and lemon essential oils in the bottle, screw on the top, and shake vigorously for 2 minutes to blend. Label the bottle and set it in a cool, dark location for 24 hours so that the oils can synergize.

Store at room temperature, away from heat and light; use within 2 years. Do not store the bottle with a dropper top, as the strong vapors will degrade the rubber tip. Store only with a screw cap.

TO DIFFUSE THE ESSENTIAL OILS: Shake well before using. Follow the manufacturer's directions for your brand of diffuser or nebulizer.

TO MAKE A SPRAY: Add 30 drops of the blend to a 4-ounce plastic or dark glass spray bottle. Then add ¼ cup of water and ¼ cup of unflavored vodka. Screw the top on the bottle and shake vigorously to blend. Label the bottle and allow the spray to synergize for 1 hour. Store at room temperature, away from heat and light; use within 1 year. Shake well before using. To take the edge off a crazy life and instill a sense of clarity, lightly mist your surrounding area and breathe deeply. Use as desired.

14 Additional Essentials

MAKES ¼ OUNCE (7.5 ML)

Cracked Skin Rescue Balm

Looking for a cracked-skin remedy with an incredibly creamy texture that melts at body temperature and penetrates amazingly well? This is the one for you. It has all the conditioning benefits of lanolin, without the odd smell, stickiness, and potential irritation, plus it's vegan! It is mildly antiseptic, anti-inflammatory, and vulnerary (skin regenerative). *Safe for folks 2 years of age and older.*

ESSENTIAL OIL

10 ◆ myrrh

BASE

4 tablespoons castor oil

2 tablespoons cocoa butter

2 tablespoons refined shea butter*

4-ounce dark glass or plastic jar

*Unrefined shea butter will work, but its stronger fragrance will greatly reduce the already subtle aroma of the essential oil, though not its properties.

TO MAKE THE BALM: Combine the castor oil, cocoa butter, and shea butter in a small saucepan over low heat, or in a double boiler, and warm until the solids are just melted. Remove from the heat and allow to cool for 5 to 10 minutes. Stir a few times to blend the mixture thoroughly. Add the myrrh essential oil directly to the jar, then slowly pour in the oil mixture. Gently stir to blend. Cap, label, and set aside until the balm has thickened, which may take up to 24 hours.

TO USE: Massage a dab of the balm into your feet, hands, shins, elbows, knees, or anywhere your skin is extremely dry, at least twice daily to seal in moisture.

Bonus uses: This formula makes a wonderful conditioner for dry, brittle nails and ragged cuticles. Simply massage a tiny bit into each nail nightly. It also can be used as a winter-weather facial shield during extreme outdoor exposure to protect your face, or as a comforting treatment for a red, raw nose while you're suffering from a bad cold.

Soothing Myrrh-Mint Mouthwash and Gargle

With a combination of warm, resinous notes and stimulating, sharp mint, this bracing, mouth-tingling blend offers antibacterial, astringent, analgesic, and anti-inflammatory properties that tone and tighten gum tissue, neutralize bad breath, soothe a sore throat, relieve laryngitis, and aid in healing mouth ulcers and inflamed gums. It is tasty and effective! *Safe for folks 12 years of age and older.*

ESSENTIAL OILS

1 ● myrrh

1 ● peppermint

BASE

¼ teaspoon sea salt

¼ cup purified water, hot or tepid (hot water is more soothing for sore throats and laryngitis)

TO MAKE THE MOUTHWASH: Combine the sea salt with the drops of myrrh and peppermint essential oils in a small mug. Pour in the water and stir to blend. Use immediately.

TO USE: Rinse your mouth thoroughly, then gargle with half of the mouthwash for up to 30 seconds (or for as long as you can tolerate). Spit it out in the sink (do not swallow). Repeat with remaining mouthwash. If you are suffering from a sore throat or laryngitis, mouth ulcers, bleeding gums, or pyorrhea, repeat several times per day until the condition improves, making a new batch each time.

MAKES ENOUGH FOR 1 USE

14 Additional Essentials

Hydrating Facial Mist

All skin types can become parched for myriad reasons: exposure to the elements (including indoor heating and air-conditioning), side effects of medication, dehydration, a poor-quality diet, and excess stress. This simple, nourishing, hydrating mist produces a cool, moist sensation on the skin, quickly quenching its thirst while calming any irritation. I've included a hint of soothing oil to boost skin's suppleness. *Safe for folks 6 years of age and older.*

ESSENTIAL OILS

8 ◆ myrrh

6 ◆ geranium

6 ◆ lavender

BASE

½ cup commercially prepared aloe vera juice

½ teaspoon vegetable glycerin

½ teaspoon almond, jojoba, extra-virgin olive, or sunflower oil

4-ounce plastic or dark glass spritzer bottle

TO MAKE THE SPRAY: Combine the myrrh, geranium, and lavender essential oils in the bottle, then add the aloe vera juice, glycerin, and your base oil of choice. Screw the top on the bottle and shake vigorously to blend. Label the bottle, set it in the refrigerator, and allow the blend to synergize for 1 hour.

Store in the refrigerator, where it will keep for up to 6 months; if you opt to keep it at room temperature, use within 4 weeks.

TO USE: Shake well, then lightly mist your skin as often as needed.

Bonus use: This blend doubles as a gentle facial toner to be used after cleansing and prior to applying moisturizer.

Eczema Relief Remedy Oil

This formula is designed specifically for those who suffer from intensely itchy eczema, be it weeping or dry. Additionally, it will deliver welcome relief to painful inflammation, reduce the redness, and stimulate the formation of new, healthy skin cells. *Safe for folks 12 years of age and older. For children aged 6 to 11, reduce the essential oils by half. For infants and children up to age 6, omit the essential oils and use only the calendula- and plantain-infused oils.*

ESSENTIAL OILS

4 ◆ German chamomile

4 ◆ myrrh

2 ◆ geranium

2 ◆ lavender

BASE

1 tablespoon calendula-infused oil (page 211)

1 tablespoon plantain-infused oil (page 212)

1-ounce dark glass bottle with a dropper top

TO MAKE THE OIL: Combine the chamomile, myrrh, geranium, and lavender essential oils in the bottle, then add the calendula and plantain oils. Screw the top on the bottle and shake vigorously for 2 minutes to blend. Label the bottle and set it in a cool, dark location for 24 hours so that the oils can synergize.

Store at room temperature, away from heat and light; use within 1 year.

TO USE: Shake well before using. With your fingertips, smooth gently over affected areas several times per day. If your eczema persists or tends to recur, please see your health-care provider.

Bonus use: To speed the healing of cuts, scrapes, bug bites or stings, or newly bruised skin, apply this oil to the affected area two or three times per day.

14 Additional Essentials

MAKES 1 OUNCE (30 ML)

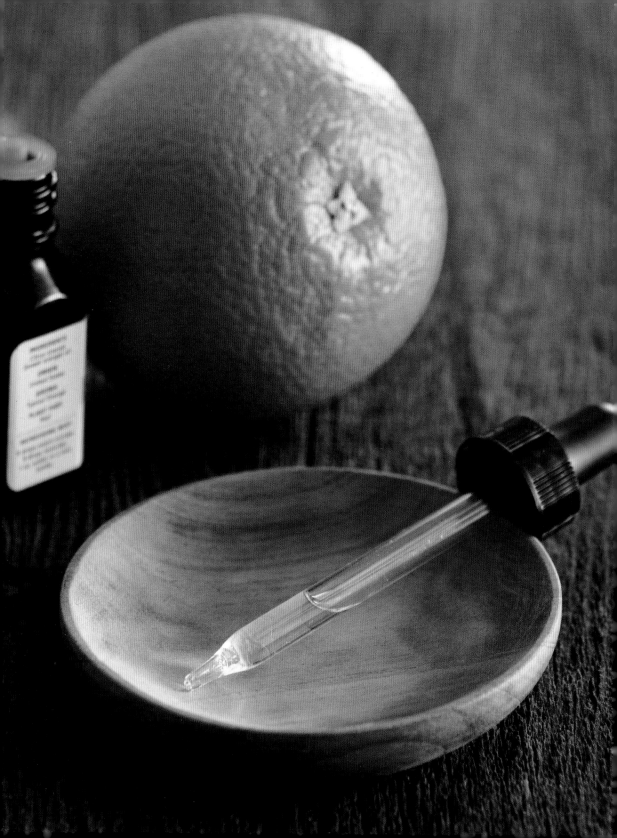

SWEET
Orange
(Citrus sinensis)

Pleasingly sweet and zesty, oranges are among the oldest cultivated fruits and were mentioned in ancient Chinese literature as long ago as 2400 BCE. The dried peel of both bitter and sweet oranges has been used in traditional Chinese medicine for thousands of years to treat anorexia, coughs, colds, malignant breast sores, cystic breasts, respiratory congestion, digestive spasms, stagnant digestion, and constipation. Throughout history, the fresh juice and oil from the pressed peel have offered valuable protection against infectious diseases as well.

Depending on the individual, sweet orange essential oil can be either relaxing or gently energizing. For most children, it acts as an aromatically pleasing sedative for the nervous system — great for use with hyperactive kids or at bedtime. But for many adults, I've noticed, it simply puts them in a good mood, instilling a sense of refreshment and revitalization. This is my oil of choice for diffusing in the morning; it starts my day off on a cheery, sunny, happy note.

One of my favorite ways to utilize the digestive benefits of orange essential oil is in synergy with peppermint oil in a massage oil blend. When combined, they are quite effective at relieving constipation, cramping, and gas. When using it in a massage oil blend for anything to do with the digestive system, remember to massage the belly in a clockwise direction, beginning at the navel and spiraling outward, ending at the top of the left thigh, to encourage the digestive process to move in the normal direction.

The astringent and toning action of orange essential oil is most beneficial for oily skin or scalp, congested skin (cystic acne or breasts), and cellulite. Orange improves the sluggish or stagnant flow of sebum (oil) and lymph within the body.

PSYCHOLOGICAL BENEFITS: A bright, cheerful oil, sweet orange lifts the spirits and instills a sense of joyfulness. It helps ease depression, improve your mood, open the heart, and reduce anxiety, irritability, restlessness, nervous tension, and other stress-related conditions, including PMS. Like other citrus oils, it builds your sense of humor and general feeling of well-being. Its calming and balancing properties help you unwind and relax, no matter how chaotic your day.

SAFETY DATA: Nontoxic, nonirritating, and generally nonsensitizing, with only a low risk of photosensitivity.

FROM HERB TO OIL

The evergreen orange tree features a rounded crown of plentiful twigs, glossy oval leaves, fragrant white flowers, and medium-size orange fruits. Thought to be native to southwestern China, it is extensively cultivated in the United States (California and Florida), the Mediterranean region, Brazil, Italy, Spain, and Israel. Much of the essential oil is produced in the United States, Brazil, Israel, Spain, and Cyprus.

The essential oil is cold-expressed from the outer peel of the ripe or almost ripe fresh fruit. It is a yellowish-orange or dark orange liquid with that familiar rich, lively aroma. Oil distilled from the peel and remains of the fruit after making juice is of inferior quality and used primarily to flavor soft drinks. Sweet orange essential oil oxidizes quickly (as do all citrus oils), so use it within 1 year, or 2 years if you keep it refrigerated.

ESSENTIAL INFORMATION

Antibacterial; gently warming; soothing and uplifting in times of stress; wonderful for use with children; fabulous flavoring for toothpastes and lip balms; deodorizing; cleansing; carminative and digestive; astringent

Happy Home, Healthy Home Blend

The uplifting, fresh, clean, light aroma of citrus essential oils makes me smile. Any stress just melts away! If you want your home to be a welcoming, comforting, healthy place for friends and family, diffusing citrus essential oils will help you create that ambience. If you adore citrus, feel free to adjust the recipe by utilizing other citrus essential oils, such as lime or tangerine.

ESSENTIAL OILS

50 ♦ sweet orange

40 ♦ grapefruit

30 ♦ bergamot

30 ♦ lemon

¼-ounce dark glass bottle with a screw cap or orifice reducer cap

TO MAKE THE BLEND: Combine the orange, grapefruit, bergamot, and lemon essential oils in the bottle. Screw the top on the bottle and shake vigorously for 2 minutes to blend. Label the bottle and set it in a cool, dark location for 24 hours so that the oils can synergize.

   Store at room temperature, away from heat and light; use within 2 years. Do not store the bottle with a dropper top, as the strong vapors will degrade the rubber tip. Store only with a screw cap.

TO DIFFUSE THE ESSENTIAL OILS: Shake well before using. Follow the manufacturer's directions for your particular brand of essential oil diffuser or nebulizer, and use the appropriate number of drops.

TO MAKE A SPRAY: Add 30 drops of the blend to a 4-ounce plastic or dark glass spray bottle. Then add ¼ cup of water and ¼ cup of unflavored vodka. Screw the top on the bottle and shake vigorously to blend. Label the bottle and allow the spray to synergize for 1 hour. Store at room temperature, away from heat and light; use within 1 year. Shake well before using. As desired, spray throughout the house and inhale the fresh, fruity aroma.

Caution: Do not use in small rooms or bedrooms with children under 2 years of age.

14 Additional Essentials

MAKES ¼ OUNCE (7.5 ML)

Sweet Orange–Mint Toothpaste

Here's a totally natural toothpaste that delivers salty-sweet flavors combined with warming and cooling sensations. It's guaranteed to tantalize your tongue and taste buds! Offering myriad benefits, this thick toothpaste helps whiten teeth and remove plaque, counters excess acid in the mouth, and freshens breath. Good stuff! For sanitary reasons, make a jar for each member of your household. *Best for folks 12 years of age and older. Due to the sodium content and gritty texture, it may irritate sensitive teeth and gums.*

ESSENTIAL OILS

15 ◊ sweet orange

10 ◊ peppermint

BASE

¼ cup baking soda

¼ cup very finely ground sea salt

2 tablespoons vegetable glycerin

2 tablespoons unrefined coconut oil

4-ounce dark glass or plastic jar

TO MAKE THE TOOTHPASTE: Combine the baking soda and salt in a small bowl. Mix well, then slowly stir in the vegetable glycerin, followed by the coconut oil. (If the coconut oil is solid or semisolid, simply set the container in a shallow pan of hot water to liquefy; it melts quickly. Or scoop the 2 tablespoons into a glass custard cup and microwave on high for a few seconds.) Stir until the mixture has a thick, creamy-granular consistency. Add the orange and peppermint essential oils, a drop at a time, stirring constantly, ensuring that they are thoroughly incorporated. Transfer the toothpaste to the jar, cap, and label. Allow toothpaste to rest for 24 hours so flavors can mingle and mellow.

Store the container away from heat and sunlight. For best flavor and texture, use within 2 months.

TO USE: Apply a small amount of paste onto your wet toothbrush and brush as normal. Do not swallow.

Orange-Honey-Cream Moisturizing Bath

Imagine the familiar, smooth, fruity scent of orange peel softened by sweet honey and the essence of rich cream. Ahhh . . . just the thought of slipping into a tub filled with this skin-pampering blend is enough to instill a bit of tranquility and make you feel pampered! Am I right? The aroma of sweet orange and calming lavender soothes the senses, while honey and cream — natural moisturizers — nourish your skin. It the perfect way to end a hectic day, and it's guaranteed to comfort and calm irritable young ones as well. Indulge, won't you? *Safe for folks 2 years of age and older.*

ESSENTIAL OILS
5 ◆ sweet orange

3 ◆ lavender

BASE
¼ cup honey, preferably raw

½ cup heavy cream, preferably organic (you can substitute light cream, half-and-half, or full-fat coconut milk)

TO MAKE THE BATH: Fill the tub with warm water. Meanwhile, combine the honey, cream, and orange and lavender essential oils in a small bowl. Stir well.

TO USE: Add the mixture to the tub and swish with your hands to thoroughly disperse the ingredients. Step in and soak for 20 to 30 minutes. When you're finished, pat your skin damp-dry and apply your favorite natural lotion or cream, if desired.

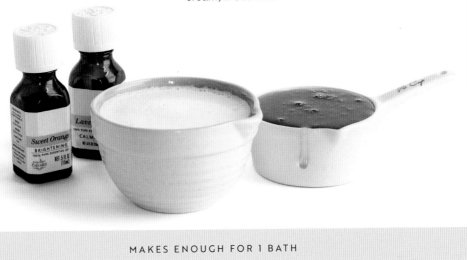

MAKES ENOUGH FOR 1 BATH

Calm, Cool, and Collected Sniffy Stick

With a gentle, lightly sweet floral-citrus-resinous aroma, this inhaler blend helps restore balance and settle a frayed spirit. You'll find it deeply soothing, centering, and grounding. *Safe for folks 12 years of age and older. For children ages 6 to 11, reduce the essential oils by half.*

ESSENTIAL OILS

8 ◆ sweet orange

6 ◆ lavender

4 ◆ Roman chamomile

4 ◆ myrrh

2 ◆ frankincense CO_2

Reusable nasal inhaler tube

TO MAKE THE SNIFFY STICK: Remove the cotton inhaler wick from the inhaler tube. Add the essential oils, drop by drop, directly to the wick. Replace the wick in the tube and tightly cap the bottom with the plug. Place the inhaler tube inside its cover and screw tightly to close; add a tiny label. To recharge, simply add more drops to the wick when the scent weakens.

Store at room temperature; for maximum potency, use within 2 to 3 months.

TO USE: Inhale deeply as needed, up to several times per day. For best results, be sure to exhale through your mouth, not your nose.

Sweet Slumber's Bliss Roll-On

Suffer from occasional insomnia? Let this gentle, citrusy-floral blend relax your mind and body and be your guide to a deep, restful night's sleep. Sweet orange, lavender, and Roman chamomile combine to make a soft, blissful aroma. *Safe for folks 6 years of age and older. For children ages 2 to 5, you may massage a little bit onto their feet.*

ESSENTIAL OILS

- 8 ◦ sweet orange
- 4 ◦ lavender
- 2 ◦ Roman chamomile

BASE

- 2 teaspoons jojoba or fractionated coconut oil

  10 ml roller-ball applicator bottle

TO MAKE THE BLEND: Combine the orange, lavender, and chamomile essential oils in the bottle, then add your base oil of choice. Cap and shake vigorously for 2 minutes. Label the bottle and set it in a cool, dark location for 24 hours so that the oils can synergize.

Store at room temperature, away from heat and light; use within 2 years.

TO USE: Shake well before each use. An hour or so before bed, and again when you climb under the covers, roll a little oil onto each temple, the base of the neck, the upper lip, and the chest. Massage in well. Next, roll some onto one palm, rub your palms together to warm the oil, then close your eyes and inhale the vapors from your cupped hands. Breathe slowly and deeply for a few minutes. Avoid direct contact with the eyes, nose, and mouth. Repeat if you wake up during the night.

14 Additional Essentials

MAKES 10 ML

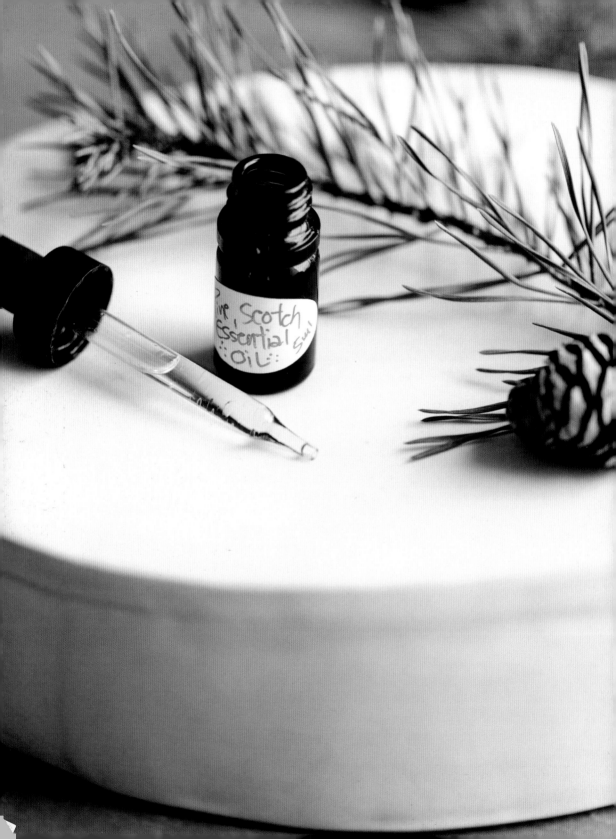

Scotch Pine

(Pinus sylvestris)

I call pine trees the "feel-good trees" because they offer so many benefits. Many of the more than 100 species of pines have been used medicinally throughout the world by cultures ranging from the Greeks, Egyptians, and Arabians to the Native Americans and Scandinavians. The needles have been burned to clear away respiratory infections and insects and stuffed into mattresses to repel lice and fleas and fend off rheumatism. The twigs were mixed with cedar and juniper for use as a purification incense.

The sticky pitch or resin that often exudes from injuries to the tree's trunk and larger limbs contains a concentration of the essential oil (as does the sap from the fir tree) and has been utilized to heal cracked skin, eczema, psoriasis, and infected wounds, and to bind cuts. Infused into a base oil as a massage oil and/or bath oil, it relieves arthritis, rheumatism, gout, sore or stiff muscles, sciatica, poor circulation of the arms and legs, chest complaints, and exhaustion. I employ this refreshing, comforting, "essence of the forest" essential oil to treat many of these conditions.

Scotch pine is considered by many aromatherapists to be one of the safest and most useful pine oils for therapeutic use, and it is the pine oil of choice for easing respiratory infections and related illnesses. Other species that I occasionally use, but which can be limited in availability, include the eastern white pine (*P. strobus*), sea pine (*P. pinaster*), and the pinyon pine (*P. edulis*).

PSYCHOLOGICAL BENEFITS: Naturally refreshing and uplifting, strengthening, empowering, and grounding, Scotch pine helps you feel open and aware. It dispels negative emotions and brings strength and comfort when you are feeling weak, unworthy, unsure, or sad. It is an excellent choice when you are experiencing nervous exhaustion and extreme fatigue as a result of stress.

SAFETY DATA: Generally nontoxic and nonirritating (except in concentration), with possible dermal sensitization to those with highly sensitive skin. Scotch pine essential oil has a rather short shelf life because it oxidizes quickly, so use it within 1 year or keep it refrigerated and use within 2 years.

Native Americans brewed pine needle tea, which is rich in vitamin C, to help prevent scurvy.

FROM HERB TO OIL

Indigenous to northern Europe and Asia and introduced to North America by European settlers, this tall conifer has deeply fissured, reddish-brown bark, long, stiff needles that grow in pairs, and pointed brown cones. It has long been cultivated in the eastern United States and Canada, mostly for Christmas tree production and as a landscape planting. The essential oil is produced primarily in the United States, Bosnia, France, Hungary, Scotland, Russia, and Austria. A colorless or pale yellow liquid with a strong, fresh, clean turpentine-like aroma, the essential oil is steam-distilled from the fresh twigs and needles. An inferior essential oil is produced by dry distillation from chipped wood and stump grindings.

ESSENTIAL PROPERTIES

Has an affinity for the respiratory tract, being a powerful antiseptic, decongestant, and expectorant; purifying and cleansing; warming circulatory stimulant that is good for pain relief; promotes healing of wounds and dry, cracked skin; deodorant; effective parasiticide against scabies and lice; strengthening, fortifying, and energizing, emotionally and physically

Herbal Analgesic Rub

I formulated this beautiful deep amber-red blend specifically to relieve arthritis flare-ups and general achiness in my own fingers, wrists, and feet, but it can also be used to ease the pain resulting from sore muscles, torn ligaments, sciatica, bruises, upper shoulder and neck tension, gout, bunions, spinal injuries, and carpal tunnel syndrome. It serves as an effective anti-inflammatory that greatly improves circulation, as well. *Safe for folks 12 years of age and older. For children aged 6 to 11, reduce the essential oils by half.*

ESSENTIAL OILS

14 ◆ Scotch pine

6 ◆ clove

2 ◆ German chamomile

2 ◆ peppermint

BASE

¼ cup St. John's wort–infused oil (page 213)

2-ounce dark glass bottle with a dropper top

TO MAKE THE RUB: Combine the pine, clove, chamomile, and peppermint essential oils in the bottle, then add the St. John's wort oil. Screw the top on the bottle and shake vigorously for 2 minutes to blend. Label the bottle and set it in a cool, dark location for 24 hours so that the oils can synergize.

Store at room temperature, away from heat and light; use within 1 year.

TO USE: Shake well before using. To ease pain, apply to affected area three or four times per day.

MAKES 2 OUNCES (60 ML)

Therapeutic "Achy Hands" Soak

Are your hands abused or overworked from the daily grind of life? Do you suffer from minor to moderate arthritis? When your hands and wrists experience aches, pains, and stiffness, for whatever reason, an old-fashioned Epsom salt hand bath infused with essential oils may be just the thing to improve comfort, circulation, and flexibility. I prefer to take this hand bath in the evening after my chores are completed, as the rich, earthy, sweet, piney scent of this blend drains the day's tensions and leaves me with a pair of very happy hands! *Safe for folks 6 years of age and older.*

ESSENTIAL OILS

3 ● Scotch pine

2 ● lavender

2 ● sweet marjoram

BASE

¼ cup Epsom salt

TO MAKE AND USE THE SOAK: Fill a basin or bowl large enough to hold both your hands and cover your wrists with water as hot as you can tolerate. Combine the Epsom salt with the Scotch pine, lavender, and marjoram essential oils in a small bowl, such as a custard cup, and stir to blend. Add to the hot water and mix thoroughly to disperse. Immerse your hands up to the wrist and soak for 10 to 20 minutes, or until the water begins to become lukewarm. Dry your hands and apply your favorite lotion or cream.

Bonus use: For achy feet, follow the directions above, but increase the amount of Epsom salt to ½ cup. Fill a foot tub or large basin with water as hot as you can tolerate. Soak your feet and ankles for 10 to 20 minutes, or until the water begins to become lukewarm. Dry your feet and apply your favorite lotion or cream.

Ease-the-Wheeze Sniffy Stick

Here's a recipe for an effective, convenient, drug-free respiratory inhaler. The essential oils, with antiviral, anti-inflammatory, antibacterial, and mucolytic properties, do an amazing job of relieving your coughing, sneezing, stuffy nose, and lung congestion. They help open and clear respiratory channels, while thinning mucus. *Safe for folks 12 years of age and older.*

ESSENTIAL OILS

- 6 ◆ eucalyptus (species *globulus*, *radiata*, or *smithii*)
- 6 ◆ Scotch pine
- 4 ◆ balsam fir
- 4 ◆ cedarwood
- 4 ◆ rosemary (ct. verbenon or nonchemotype specific)

Reusable nasal inhaler

TO MAKE THE SNIFFY STICK: Remove the cotton inhaler wick from the inhaler tube. Add the essential oils, drop by drop, directly to the wick. Replace the wick in the tube and tightly cap the bottom with the plug. Place the inhaler tube inside its cover and screw tightly to close; add a tiny label. To recharge, simply add more drops to the wick when the scent weakens.

Store at room temperature; for maximum potency, use within 2 to 3 months.

TO USE: Inhale deeply through your nose, up to several times per day. For best results, be sure to exhale through your mouth, not your nose. If you're too congested to inhale through your nose, then inhale and exhale through your mouth. The formula will still be absorbed and distributed throughout your body.

Bonus use: To fend off illness, use this aromatic stick as a great immune booster during cold and flu season.

Caution: If you suffer from asthma, this formulation may be too stimulating. Avoid completely if you are having an asthma attack.

"Breathe Free" Herbal Vapor Rub

This blend contains strong respiratory antiseptics to help fight infection and mucolytics to aid in dissolving and loosening mucous congestion. Decongestant, antiviral, and analgesic properties help heal the source of your stuffiness, relieve sinus headaches, shrink swollen mucous membranes, and alleviate tightness in your lungs. Potent aromatherapy, indeed! *Safe for folks 12 years of age and older. This is an aromatherapeutically concentrated formula, so use only as directed.*

ESSENTIAL OILS

25 ◆ Scotch pine

20 ◆ balsam fir

20 ◆ eucalyptus (species *globulus*, *radiata*, or *smithii*)

10 ◆ lavender

10 ◆ peppermint

5 ◆ clove

5 ◆ tea tree

5 ◆ thyme (ct. linalool or nonchemotype specific)

BASE

½ cup almond, jojoba, extra-virgin olive, or sunflower oil

4-ounce dark glass bottle with a dropper top

TO MAKE THE RUB: Combine the pine, balsam fir, eucalyptus, lavender, peppermint, clove, tea tree, and thyme essential oils in the bottle, then add your base oil of choice. Screw the top on the bottle and shake vigorously for 2 minutes to blend. Label the bottle and set it in a cool, dark location for 24 hours so that the oils can synergize.

Store at room temperature, away from heat and light; use within 1 year (or 2 years if you used jojoba oil).

TO USE: Shake well before using. Apply a drop or two of oil under your nose, on your throat, on your temples, behind your ears, and on your chest. If your skin is not too sensitive, place a drop on each cheekbone as well. Apply a few drops to the soles of your feet. Massage the oil completely into your skin, then cup your hands over your mouth and nose, close your eyes, and inhale the essences. Inhale through your mouth if your nose is congested. Avoid direct contact with the eyes, nose, and mouth. Repeat several times per day.

"Breathe Free" Herbal Steam

Having similar actions and properties as the "Breathe Free" Herbal Vapor Rub, this recipe is a steaming vapors alternative that provides relief for respiratory congestion. I swear by this steam when I have a bad head cold or sinus head-ache, or when my lungs feel heavy and congested. It really helps drain away the misery and seems to open up everything! A bonus: the stimulating aroma leaves your house smelling ultra-fresh and clean. *Safe for folks 12 years of age and older.*

ESSENTIAL OILS

2 ◆ Scotch pine

1 ◆ eucalyptus (species *globulus* or *radiata*)

1 ◆ balsam fir or Scotch pine

BASE

3 cups purified water

Caution: Do not use if you suffer from asthma, if you have sensitive skin, or if you are experiencing any type of skin irritation.

TO MAKE AND USE THE STEAM: Bring water to just shy of a boil and pour into a large heat-proof bowl. Place the bowl on a stable surface, in a location where you can either stand or sit comfortably for 5 to 10 minutes. Add the essential oils and swish the water to disperse them a bit.

Immediately drape a large bath towel over your head, neck, shoulders, and the steaming bowl to create a vapor tent. With your eyes closed and your face 8 to 12 inches from the surface of the water, breathe deeply and relax. If your nose is clogged, inhale through your mouth. You should begin to sweat and your nose should run — that's a good thing. Your circulation is moving. If you begin to feel uncomfortable, pop your head out of the tent for a few moments of fresh air, then go right back in. Keep your eyes closed during the entire steam.

When you're finished, splash your face and neck with tepid water, followed by a few splashes of cool water. Pat your skin almost dry and follow with an application of light moisturizer, if desired. You may partake of this treatment once or twice per day until you are feeling better.

14 Additional Essentials

5

The Essential Home Apothecary

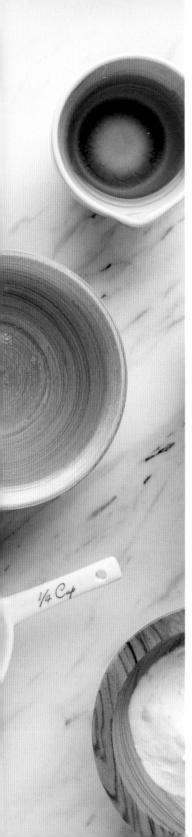

In this section, you'll find a comprehensive guide to the base and infused oils, thickeners, blending liquids, and other plant-based constituents used in the recipes in this book. Following the ingredient descriptions is a list of the necessary kitchen equipment and packaging supplies. Please use this handy guide as an educational reference as you create and concoct your own essential oil products.

If this is your first foray into making these types of remedies, some of the ingredients may seem foreign. "Where the heck do I find all this stuff?" you might wonder. Don't worry, most of these items are readily available. Start by looking at your local health food store, food co-op, or whole foods grocer; the Internet, of course, is a go-to resource for *everything* you'll need to create all the recipes in this book. I tend to purchase from mail-order catalogs or Internet sources that I know have a relatively rapid turnover of stock, so I can be sure the ingredients I purchase are fresh. (For a listing of my trusted suppliers, see page 229.)

Base Oils

Base oils are chemically classified as fats — they contain fatty acids and glycerin — and are derived from beans, nuts, seeds, fruits, and grains. You may also hear them called carrier oils, unctuous oils, or fixed oils. Base oils are characteristically slippery to the touch, smooth in texture, and lighter than water, with an extremely low evaporation rate. They leave a permanent grease spot when dropped on paper, unlike essential oils, which evaporate with little trace.

Base oils are used as carrying agents. When combined with herbs and warmed for a period of time, base oils are efficient solvents for extracting and absorbing the herbs' fat-soluble chemical constituents. Combining the oils with essential oils is a shortcut to this extraction; the base oil in this case simply carries the essential oil into the skin. A wonderful benefit derived from using base oils infused with plants or their extracts in topical remedies is that as they are absorbed, they leave behind a protective, skin-conditioning barrier on the surface while delivering the herbal benefits to the tissues below. I use only plant-derived fats — never lanolin, lard, cod liver oil, or mineral oil — as I find plant oils to be completely biocompatible with the skin, triggering very few skin sensitivities and having no objectionable odors. See page 225 for more information on making and using herbal infused oils.

The best base oils are organically grown, naturally extracted, and minimally processed. The key words to look for on the label are *organic, cold pressed, expeller pressed,* and/or *unrefined* — these generally guarantee the highest quality. Unrefined, organic oils that were either expeller pressed or cold pressed are the most desirable. These oils have not been exposed to extraction procedures using petroleum-derived solvents such as hexane (one of the most common), nor to extremely high heat, bleaching, or deodorizing. These processes can destroy or alter an oil's natural molecular state, thereby affecting aromas, flavors, colors, consistency, and antioxidant properties, plus the vitamin, mineral, and essential fatty acid content.

More gently processed oils are produced by mechanically pressing beans, fruits, nuts, seeds, or grains and straining out any resulting debris. Some heat is naturally generated during the pressing; the oil usually reaches a temperature of between 80° and 175°F (27° and 79°C), which is not so hot that it destroys the vital nutrients, taste, and aroma of the oil. Compared to their refined, highly processed cousins (which are commonly found in the average supermarket), unrefined organic oils often appear slightly darker in color, are truer to taste, have deeper aromas, and contain much higher amounts of essential fatty acids. They may also at times have a cloudy appearance.

Storing Base Oils

It's important to note that most unrefined base oils — with the exception of avocado, coconut, extra-virgin olive, jojoba, and sesame — have a relatively short shelf life and tend to become rancid if stored at room temperature for more than 8 months, especially in warm weather. These oils should be refrigerated and used within 1 year. As a rule, I refrigerate all of my base oils, except jojoba, extra-virgin olive, and coconut, which are exceptionally stable. These I store in a cool, dark cabinet.

If you purchase an oil that has a strange "off" smell, then it's probably rancid and should be returned to where you bought it. (But note that certain oils — especially those that are organic and unrefined — such as macadamia, apricot kernel, tamanu, hemp, hazelnut, sesame, coconut, and extra-virgin olive — naturally have strong fragrances.) Purchase base oils from reputable retailers with a high turnover of inventory, and *always* check the expiration date on the bottle.

Recommended Base Oils

Each base oil used in my recipes has individual characteristics that I take into consideration, such as texture, weight, slip (how it glides or flows on the skin), fragrance, ability to penetrate the skin, and shelf life, which determine how it is blended and its intended purpose. There is indeed a method to my madness! Kitchen chemistry is a fun art learned over time, and I encourage you to explore its many facets.

Almond Oil, Sweet
(Prunus dulcis)
Pressed from the ripened kernel, this is an all-purpose, nutritious, very emollient, light- to medium-weight pale golden oil with a neutral to slightly warming energy. High in monounsaturated fatty acids, it

penetrates and conditions the skin. It is recommended for all skin types, but especially dry, inflamed, or itchy skin.

Castor Oil
(Ricinus communis)
This shiny, viscous, clear to pale amber-gold oil is processed from the beans of an annual shrub. It's highly emollient and analgesic and has a warming energy; it is frequently used topically to help relieve minor arthritic pain and muscle spasms, to stimulate lymph movement, and to break down dense, fibrous tissue. Castor oil is the primary oil in most creamy and glossy lipsticks on the commercial market, and it provides staying power and shine to natural lip balm and gloss recipes. It's particularly good

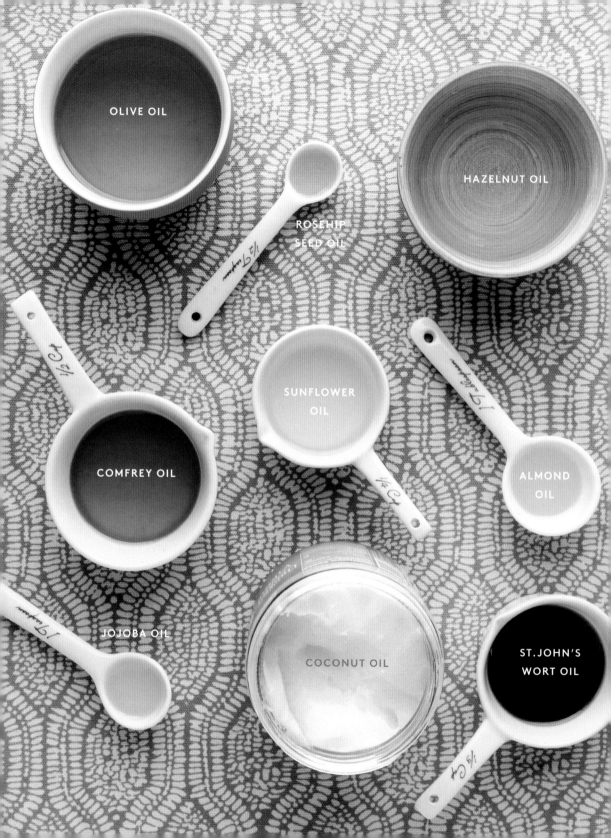

OLIVE OIL

HAZELNUT OIL

ROSEHIP
SEED OIL

SUNFLOWER
OIL

COMFREY OIL

ALMOND
OIL

JOJOBA OIL

COCONUT OIL

ST. JOHN'S
WORT OIL

for softening rough, dry skin on the heels, knees, and elbows and patches of eczema and psoriasis, plus it works fabulously and inexpensively as a diaper rash and foot-blister preventive. When applied to fingernails and cuticles, it shields against the drying effects of detergents, hot water, and dry winter air.

Coconut Oil
(*Cocos nucifera*)

I prefer to use only unrefined organic, cold-pressed, virgin coconut oil. Its sweet, exotic fragrance and smooth flavor are reminiscent of a tropical paradise (in contrast, refined coconut oil is void of both fragrance and flavor). Coconut oil is derived from the fruit of the coconut palm and is solid at temperatures below 76°F (24°C).

It is highly emollient and an excellent oil for all-over use — some people swear by it as the ultimate skin softener, hair conditioner, and after-sun treatment. Use this tasty, anti-inflammatory, energetically cooling oil in natural toothpastes, lip balms, dry skin and scalp conditioning oils, baby oils, cold sore treatments, or any oil-based product from which you desire a penetrating, softening effect. It makes the perfect intimate lubricant, too, though it is not latex friendly.

Fractionated coconut oil, sometimes called "liquid coconut oil," is a form of refined coconut oil that has had its long-chain fatty acids removed. This change alone makes the oil liquid at room temperature and extends the product's shelf life. It is odorless, very light in texture, and highly penetrating; the skin absorbs it quickly. It leaves skin feeling soft and smooth, not greasy, and it won't exacerbate oiliness, though it may aggravate acne-prone skin. I often offer it as an alternative to jojoba oil when creating formulations to be applied with a roller-ball bottle, especially those for the face or neck.

Jojoba
(*Simmondsia chinensis*)

Pronounced *ho-ho-ba,* this light- to medium-textured oil (technically a liquid wax ester) is derived from the seeds of a desert shrub that is cultivated in the southwestern United States, Argentina, and Israel. Chemically similar to the natural restorative esters produced by our skin's sebaceous glands, with a neutral to slightly warming energy, top-quality jojoba oil contains alpha, delta, and gamma tocopherols, all natural forms of the antioxidant vitamin E. It also serves as a mild anti-inflammatory agent. It's one of my favorite base oils because it penetrates extremely well, leaves no oily residue, does not turn rancid, requires no refrigeration, and is great for *all* skin types. Jojoba is my primary choice when making treatments for thinning hair, alopecia, scalp disorders, and cradle cap.

Olive Oil, Extra-Virgin
(Olea europaea)

This rich, relatively stable, moderately heavy green oil, derived from the first pressing of ripe and unripe olives, has a strong olive aroma and taste. It contains high levels of monounsaturated fatty acids, antioxidants, enzymes, vitamins, and minerals. In formulations, it can be used alone or blended with lighter-textured, less aromatic oils. With a neutral energy, highly emollient quality, and gently antiseptic and stimulant properties, olive oil makes a wonderful base oil for medicinal salves, infused oils, and essential oil blends, and many herbalists use it exclusively. It also makes an excellent conditioning oil for dry skin, dry nails, eczema, and psoriasis. Unrefined, unfiltered organic Tuscan olive oil is my number one favorite oil for skin care.

Rosehip Seed Oil
(Rosa rubiginosa; R. moschata)

This medium-weight, amber-red oil pressed from ripened rosehips has a light, slightly tart aroma and a neutral to warming energy. It contains extremely high levels of essential fatty acids, making it an ideal nourishing and conditioning agent for scar tissue, stretch marks, wrinkles, and weathered, dry, devitalized skin. An amazing skin-cell regenerative, anti-inflammatory, and anti-aging oil, it serves as a vegan alternative to animal-derived collagen treatments as it dramatically increases the elasticity of the skin and stimulates the formation of new collagen fibrils, resulting in a smoother, more toned appearance to the skin. I frequently combine this oil with tamanu to enhance its healing properties. Rosehip seed oil has a short shelf life of 4 to 6 months; always keep it refrigerated.

Contraindications: Avoid using rosehip seed oil on oily, acneic, or combination skin, as it may exacerbate these conditions.

Sunflower Oil
(Helianthus annuus)

Derived from the pressed seeds of the sunflower, this light- to medium-textured oil is rich in oleic acid, lecithin, minerals, and vitamins A and E. Deeply nourishing and conditioning, with a slightly sweet flavor and cooling energy, it is an all-purpose and inexpensive oil. I particularly recommend it (or jojoba) as a formulation base for those with sensitive skin who suffer from dermatitis (red, rashy, inflamed skin), skin infections, acne, eczema, or psoriasis.

Tamanu Oil
(Calophyllum inophyllum; C. tacamahaca)

This rich, brownish-green oil is also known as calophyllum or foraha oil. Derived from the ripened seeds or nuts of a tree indigenous to tropical Southeast Asia, East Africa, South India, and the Polynesian Islands, it has a sweet, earthy fragrance reminiscent of buttercream frosting or Kahlua. It's mildly analgesic, antiseptic, and anti-inflammatory, with a slightly cooling energy, and it is often used in oil blends, salves, and balms specifically formulated to help fade scars, heal burns and boils, and soothe chapped or bruised skin, eczema, psoriasis, and herpes sores. It's a perfect choice for environmentally damaged, mature, or very dry skin.

Herb-Infused Oils

As an herbalist, I never pass up the opportunity to integrate herbs into my aromatherapy formulations, and herb-infused oils most definitely pair well with essential oils. Just what is an infused oil? To *infuse* a plant means to steep or soak plant material (leaves, bark, flowers, and the like) in a menstruum (solvent) such as water, alcohol, or oil in order to extract the soluble properties of the plant. An herb-infused oil is a base oil that has absorbed the fat-soluble properties of a chosen herb that was allowed to soak in warmed oil for a period of time. When the infusion is complete, the herb matter is strained out and the resulting oil is bottled for future use.

Infused oils contain myriad healing and soothing properties. They are often used topically to comfort or remedy a health concern, but when blended with certain essential oils and allowed to synergize for up to 24 hours, they create a most harmonious healing elixir, providing enhanced medicine for your being.

Allow me to introduce you to four of my favorite gentle yet medicinally potent, amazingly useful herbs. They make wonderful infused oil. You can buy these infused oils from most herb shops, natural foods stores, or online, but making them yourself produces a fresher, and, I think, more potent result. If you are interested in creating your own herb-infused oils, from either fresh or dried herbs, consult the appendix on page 225.

Calendula
(Calendula officinalis)
The sunny calendula flower, ranging from bright yellow to deep orange, has a neutral to cooling energy and is traditionally known for its calming, anti-inflammatory, vulnerary, antiseptic, and slightly astringent properties. Calendula-infused oil, with its vibrant orange hue, promotes healthy granulation of skin tissue and rapid healing, making it especially beneficial for environmentally damaged, abraded, inflamed, itchy, cracked, chapped, dry, or infected skin.

Additionally, I recommend it for treating minor to moderate burns, sunburns, stretch marks, psoriasis and eczema, scars less than two years old, bug bites and stings, poison plant rashes, hives, shingles, and diaper rash. It conditions skin by restoring elasticity and suppleness. In formulations for children, the elderly, or those with sensitive skin, where gentle effectiveness is of utmost importance, calendula oil is an excellent choice.

To prepare for infusing: Use the entire flower, including the thick, sticky, resinous bracts that form the green base of the flower head. Allow to wilt for at least 72 hours, or use in dried form.

Comfrey
(*Symphytum officinale*)

Comfrey is a 3-foot-tall bushy perennial plant with large, deep green fuzzy leaves and small, pretty purple flowers. Both the leaves and roots have soothing, comforting, mildly astringent and antiseptic, anti-inflammatory, and vulnerary properties with a cooling energy. The root is particularly mucilaginous (slippery and gooey) and emollient. Personally, I favor the leaves for infusing into oil as they wilt or dry readily when freshly picked. The moisture-laden roots take much, much longer to lose enough moisture so that you can infuse them into oil. However, when I have access to dried root, I'll use it.

Comfrey-infused oil, applied topically on a regular basis, offers analgesic relief for muscular soreness and stiffness, strains, sprains, achy or arthritic joints, and gout. Due to comfrey's inherent skin-mending properties, it will dramatically speed cell proliferation in cases

of damaged or irritated skin, making it effective for dermatitis, poison plant rashes, minor to moderate burns, cuts and scrapes, bug bites and stings, bruises, ulcerations, hemorrhoids, scars less than two years old, and stretch marks. It is also wonderful for dry, cracked, chapped, or fissured skin.

To prepare for infusing: Allow fresh comfrey leaves to wilt for 48 to 72 hours, or used in dried form.

Contraindications: Do not use on deep cuts or puncture wounds, as the oil may stimulate the outer layer of skin tissue to mend and seal the wound before regeneration of deeper subsurface tissues, which could result in an internal infection. Use it after the wound has significantly closed.

Plantain
(*Plantago major, P. lanceolata*)

A common "weed" that grows in lawns and wastelands throughout the world, plantain has flat, spreading leaves that grow from a rosette center. It has a cold energy with vulnerary, antiseptic, anti-inflammatory, and potent astringent properties. The leaves contain a wonderful mucilaginous substance that is quite soothing for skin irritations — in fact, if you get stung by a bee and need quick relief, locate a plantain leaf, chew it to a pulp, and apply this "spit paste" to the sting. It cools and calms within minutes!

I use plantain-infused oil to treat all manner of skin irritations and infections, but it's especially effective for those that are weeping or oozing with heat or infection, such as blisters, boils, bedsores and skin ulcers, poison plant rashes, diaper rash, cuts and scrapes, hemorrhoids, and insect bites and stings. This is a superior oil for newly bruised, inflamed, swollen skin. Plantain is ever so gentle and quite effective, and it grows practically everywhere. There's nothing like "free" medicine!

To prepare for infusing: Allow fresh plantain leaves to wilt for 48 to 72 hours, or use in dried form.

St. John's Wort
(*Hypericum perforatum*)

A European native, now naturalized in North America and Australia, this invasive roadside "weed" has clusters of star-shaped, bright yellow flowers atop 2- to 3-foot-tall stems, with small leaves. The petals have tiny black dots on their back edges, which is where the medicinal hypericin constituents are stored. St. John's wort has a cooling energy and serves as a highly effective nervine, astringent, analgesic, vulnerary, antispasmodic, antiviral, and anti-inflammatory agent.

The flowers and buds make a vivid blood-red infused oil with a lovely sweet-tart aroma. I use this oil topically to treat nervous tension, bedsores and skin ulcers, hemorrhoids, sciatica, spinal injuries, bruises, headaches, cold sores, and shingles. It is wonderfully beneficial when used to treat inflamed or injured muscles, joints, and tendons, as well as nerve damage, chronic multiple sclerosis, arthritis, and gout. I frequently use both St. John's wort– and comfrey-infused oils in my reflexology practice to soothe achy feet and hands.

To prepare for infusing: The flowering and budding tops must be processed fresh, after being allowed to wilt for 24 to 48 hours. (Dried St. John's wort does not make good medicine when infused in oil.) Resist the temptation to use only the flowers and buds, which is the typical recommendation in most herb books, as the leaves contain active flavonoids that augment the healing activity of the compounds (hypericins) found in the flowers and buds. I tend to include an approximate one-eighth portion of chopped upper stems and leaves into the mix.

HARVESTING CAUTION: When you are handling the fresh herb, you can readily absorb hypericins through the skin, leading to photosensitivity, plus your hands will be stained reddish-purple, so wearing gloves is recommended. Take care not to wipe the delicate tissues around the eyes or the brow with hypericin-laden hands while harvesting, as these areas are particularly sensitive. Wash your hands well after handling the fresh herb.

Contraindication: St. John's wort topical application can lead to photosensitivity. Keep treated areas covered if you are venturing into direct sunlight.

Other Carriers and Blending Ingredients

Sometimes a base oil isn't the preferred carrier for a particular blend of essential oils, or a different medium is desired. You wouldn't want to spray oil all over yourself when a cooling alcohol base is called for, for example. Listed here are several ingredients that you may want to have on hand as you embark on your essential oil adventures.

Aloe Vera Juice
(*Aloe barbadensis*)

With its cold energy and mildly astringent, tissue-tightening, anti-inflammatory, and vulnerary properties, aloe soothes "hot" ailments such as itchy rashes, insect bites and stings, burns, bedsores and skin ulcers, eczema, pso-riasis, hemorrhoids, minor infections, blemishes, and hot flashes. An incredibly hydrating extract, aloe vera juice speeds skin cell regeneration and encourages rapid healing. Aloe gel may be used instead, but it can be rather thick and chunky, making it difficult to pour into small-necked bottles.

Baking Soda
(Sodium bicarbonate)

This white, odorless, alkaline, salty-tasting powder has skin-soothing and softening properties. It relieves the pain and itch of bee stings, rashes, and contact dermatitis; deodorizes feet and underarms; softens bath water; serves as a base for natural toothpastes and bath salts; and can help relieve acid indigestion. Inexpensive and multipurpose!

Beeswax

Secreted by worker honeybees, pure unrefined, unbleached beeswax adds a sweet fragrance and golden color to products. It is commonly used as a thickener in herbal salves, balms, creams, and lotions. Melted beeswax hardens quickly as it cools. Beeswax is available in many forms: honeycomb sheets that can be broken or cut; convenient pastilles or pellets that can be measured and melted with ease; or solid blocks and small chunks that can be placed in a ziplock freezer bag and whacked with a hammer into smaller pieces.

POSSIBLE SUBSTITUTE: Refined vegetable emulsifying wax does not have the same alluring qualities as beeswax but is a good vegan substitute. I prefer to use fresh beeswax that I obtain locally, when available, as I appreciate the skin-conditioning properties and adore the aroma.

Cocoa Butter
(*Theobroma cacao*)

Derived from roasted cocoa beans, this cream-colored, chocolaty-smelling emollient vegetable fat is hard at room temperature but melts at body temperature. It lends a thick, creamy consistency with soothing, conditioning properties for the skin. Cocoa butter is a wonderful addition to salve and balm recipes formulated for personal lubricants (though it is *not* latex friendly), pregnant bellies and expanding breasts, and the tender skin of children and the elderly. It is ever so gentle and edible, to boot! Cocoa butter is available as a solid in jars, chunks, or convenient wafers, which are easily measured and melted.

Epsom Salt
(Magnesium sulfate)

Soothe and relax with this classic bath salt. It can be used by itself or combined with essential oils for a splendid soak. In the bath or as a foot or hand soak, it relieves aches and pains and lactic acid buildup in overused, sore muscles. It's especially good for reviving tired, achy feet or soothing hard-working hands.

Glycerin, Vegetable

A natural emollient derived from vegetable fats, this clear, slippery, super-thick moisturizing liquid acts as a humectant (drawing moisture from the air to the skin) when used in small quantities in cosmetic and remedial formulations. But if it makes up more than 20 percent of a formula, it can have the opposite effect of drawing moisture from within the skin toward its surface. I add it to recipes for lip balms, lip glosses, and breath sprays for its sweet flavor and moisturizing quality, and I add it to homemade toothpastes for the smooth texture it provides. Glycerin easily dissolves into watery and alcohol-based solutions. In vodka-based formulations, it ameliorates the skin-drying effect of the alcohol.

Shea Butter
(*Vitellaria paradoxa*)

Pressed from the nuts of the karite tree, native to Africa, unrefined shea butter is a soft, cream-to-pale-gold solid fat. It often has a distinctive fragrance that's difficult to mask. If the scent displeases you, purchase the refined butter, which is slightly firmer, whiter in color, and much less aromatic. (I actually prefer shea butter in the refined form.) Shea butter contributes a thick and creamy texture with skin-softening properties when added to salves and balms. It can even be used alone. Shea butter takes much longer to harden than beeswax, so if you use it as the primary thickening agent, your product will need additional time to completely set up — sometimes up to 48 hours if the room is very warm.

Vinegar, Raw Apple Cider

Raw apple cider vinegar has a host of beneficial enzymes, vitamins, and minerals, as well as probiotics and many other health-promoting properties. But this is true only for *raw* unpasteurized cider vinegar. Vinegar that is not raw is heated to a high temperature and filtered, which destroys the beneficial enzymes, alters the vitamins and minerals, and minimizes the properties that inhibit unfriendly bacteria. I prefer Bragg organic apple cider vinegar, but there are other quality brands. Raw vinegar tastes deliciously sweet-tart and tangy and has a rich, cloudy brownish color. I employ it as a topical remedy to dissolve warts, to relieve cases of vaginitis and itchy or rashy skin, and as an immune-boosting base in my favorite Essential Four Thieves Vinegar formula (page 103).

Vitamin E Oil

This antioxidant oil, commonly derived from soybeans or sunflower seeds, acts as both a healing agent and a natural preservative in oil-based recipes such as bath and massage oils, remedial oil blends, salves, balms, and infused oils. When applied topically, it aids in the prevention of scar tissue formation and speeds healing of damaged tissue. I generally call for 1,000 IU of liquid vitamin E oil for every cup (8 ounces/240 ml) of base oil or infused oil. Using 400 IU capsules (or larger) is convenient; simply pierce the capsules and squeeze out the oil. Buy organic, if available, as most natural vitamin E oils are extracted from genetically modified or pesticide-treated plants. Look for *d-alpha tocopherol* (you may also see *mixed tocopherols*) on the label to indicate that the oil is of natural origin; *dl-alpha tocopherol* indicates that it is synthetic. The latter generally costs half as much as the natural form but is significantly less potent.

VODKA

VITAMIN E OIL

VEGETABLE
GLYCERIN

BAKING SODA

ALOE VERA
JUICE

COCOA
BUTTER

WHITE
KAOLIN
CLAY

WITCH HAZEL

UNREFINED
SHEA BUTTER

VEGETABLE
GLYCERIN

EPSOM SALT

Vodka (Ethyl Alcohol)

Commonly derived from the fermentation of grain or potatoes, this fragrance-free, antiseptic alcoholic liquid is often used as an extractive solvent for herbal tinctures to be used both orally and topically. In this book, I use plain vodka either as the primary product base or blended with water and other ingredients. Alcohol helps dissolve essential oils and hold them in solution for products such as insect repellents, air fresheners, sanitizing sprays, deodorants, breath sprays, wound washes, and liniments. Always purchase unflavored 80- or 100-proof vodka; an inexpensive brand is fine. Despite what you might read in other aromatherapy books, there's no need to purchase ethanol, which is 95 percent alcohol and not as readily available.

White Kaolin Clay

Also called white cosmetic clay, this naturally absorbent and mineral-rich powdered clay is used as a base for tooth powders and pastes, natural deodorants, body powders, and facial masks. It also makes an excellent drawing poultice for insect bites and stings, minor to moderate skin infections, and acne blemishes.

Witch Hazel
(Hamamelis virginiana)

A small, deciduous tree with stringy, bright yellow flowers, native to the damp woodlands of eastern North America and Nova Scotia, witch hazel has a neutral to cooling energy with antiseptic, anti-inflammatory, hemostatic, and astringent properties. It contains high levels of tannins, which make it quite bitter and drying, plus eugenol and carvacrol, essential oil constituents that act as stimulating, anti-infectious agents.

Many topical herbal remedies call for a witch hazel extract. Though you can find this product in any pharmacy, I recommend making your own at home (see facing page for an easy recipe), as your formula will be stronger and more effective. Alternatively, you can purchase superior witch hazel from online purveyors of herbal product ingredients. It makes a good base for insect repellent and deodorant sprays, as well as an effective treatment for boils, blisters, bruises, blemishes, hemorrhoids, minor infections, insect bites and stings, athlete's foot, contact dermatitis, and poison plant rashes.

Make Your Own Witch Hazel

Depending on the brand, most commercial versions are approximately 14 percent isopropyl alcohol (a solvent derived from petroleum-based propylene) or ethanol (made from the fermentation of starch, sugar, or other carbohydrates), and the other 86 percent is a watery extract of the plant. I think this easy recipe results in a more potent and effective anti-inflammatory astringent.

> 8 tablespoons dried witch hazel bark (or 16 tablespoons crushed fresh bark)

> 2 cups 80-proof unflavored vodka (an inexpensive brand is fine)

Combine the witch hazel and vodka in a 1-quart canning jar. Put a small piece of plastic wrap over the mouth of the jar, then screw down the lid snugly and store it in a cool, dark place for at least 8 weeks, shaking daily. The longer it sits, the stronger the final product.

Strain out the plant matter; your yield will be somewhat less than the original 2 cups, especially if you used dried bark. Stored at room temperature, away from heat and light, it will last almost indefinitely.

Mixing It Up:
Essential Equipment

The idea of making your own remedies from natural ingredients may seem a bit daunting, but it really shouldn't be. It's easy and soul-satisfying and can be a lot of fun. Only basic kitchen equipment and cooking skills, a variety of storage containers, and easy-to-follow recipes (which are in this book!) are necessary for producing wonderfully fresh, health- and wellness-nurturing creations.

An average home kitchen stocked with standard cooking implements will supply you with just about everything you need to prepare simple herbal products, and anything you don't already own should be readily available at your local home goods, department, kitchenware, or hardware store or from online purveyors of related kitchen equipment. The basics are listed on the following pages.

BOWLS. You'll need a variety of sizes in glass, enamel, plastic, stainless steel, or ceramic — no copper or aluminum, please, as they can react adversely with some of the chemical compounds in the essential oils and herbs.

CUTTING BOARD. My favorite cutting boards are flexible plastic mats, which I place atop my wooden board. They make it easy to transfer the chopped ingredients directly to the bowl, canning jar, saucepan, or double boiler. Don't process your herbs or any other ingredients on a board that is used for dairy, fish, or meat products; I recommend having one just for herbal remedies. Keep your boards or mats scrupulously clean at all times; they can harbor bacteria in grooves and scratches.

DOUBLE BOILER. A double boiler is a two-part pot designed to moderate the heat that comes directly off a stovetop burner. The bottom section holds simmering water, while the ingredients go in the top part. I occasionally use a double boiler to melt hard or thick ingredients, such as beeswax or shea butter, or to warm liquid oils when I'm making salves and balms. It is handy for making infused oils that require a low temperature. The advantage of this tool is that it produces a gentle, even, relatively low heat, making it impossible to scorch or boil your ingredients if you happen to get called away from the kitchen or get distracted. Avoid ones made from aluminum or copper, which can react negatively with the chemical compounds in essential oils and herbs.

FILTERS. I prefer paper coffee filters because they retain *all* particulate matter when you are straining herb-infused oils and liniments. I use the small or medium unbleached basket-style filters as liners for handheld mesh strainers and the bigger basket-style ones to line a pasta colander for straining larger quantities. I don't recommend the cone-style filters, as the glue sometimes dissolves, especially when it comes into contact with ethyl alcohol.

A doubled or tripled layer of cheesecloth, an old nylon stocking, a muslin bag or piece of muslin fabric, a linen seed-sprouting bag, or any finely woven mesh bag makes a good substitute, though some herbal particulate matter may filter through and then the product will require re-straining.

FUNNEL. A small one made of plastic or stainless steel makes it easier to pour liquids into narrow-necked storage bottles.

GLASS DROPPER. Sometimes called an eyedropper or a pipette, a dropper is used for measuring essential oils by the drop. Glass is preferable to plastic because it doesn't retain scent or color from the oils, and some essential oils, especially undiluted citrus oils, will rapidly degrade plastic. After each use, rinse the dropper with hot water, then pour isopropyl rubbing alcohol or 95 percent ethyl alcohol (inexpensive 80-proof vodka works great) through it to sterilize it. Allow it to thoroughly dry before using it again.

An Important Tip

Never use a dropper top to seal a bottle of undiluted essential oil. These oils are quite volatile and the vapors will rapidly degrade the rubber, allowing air to enter, diminishing the quality of your investment.

Most essential oils come in 5 ml, 10 ml, or 15 ml bottles, with "drop-by-drop" reducers for easy dispensing, eliminating the need for a dropper, but larger bottles are often sealed with a simple screw top.

MEASURING CUPS AND SPOONS. Glass, plastic, or stainless steel cups and spoons used for baking are fine.

MORTAR AND PESTLE. This rather old-fashioned herbalist's tool is handy for combining essential oils with powdered ingredients when you're making tooth powders, body powders, and clay packs. I recommend a larger model with a mortar approximately 6 inches in diameter.

POTS AND PANS. For making balms, salves, and infused oils, I use pots in several sizes made from enamel, glass, or stainless steel. Don't use aluminum or copper, which can react negatively with the chemical compounds in essential oils and herbs.

SPATULAS. Collect a variety of sizes for scooping out thick ingredients or products from any type of container. Short, narrow spatulas are useful for filling small jars with thickened salves and balms or for transferring products from one container to another.

SPOONS AND STIRRING UTENSILS. One small and one medium wooden spoon are indispensable. A stainless ice-tea or soup spoon works well for blending liquids in tiny pans or custard cups. Wooden chopsticks, thin dowels, old flatware knives and forks, and the handles of wooden spoons are useful for poking into tall containers, as well as for dredging sludgy oil-sodden herbs from saucepans, double boilers, or canning jars. A basic whisk of any material works well for blending batches of powdered ingredients with essential oils.

STRAINERS. Choose stainless steel or sturdy fabric mesh, and use them to strain herbs from liquids or to support finer filters, such as paper coffee filters or muslin, when straining smaller particles.

THERMOMETER (YOGURT OR CANDY). It's important to monitor the temperature of your herb and oil mixtures during the infusion process. Whatever type of thermometer you choose, make sure it reads temperatures that begin at the lower end of the scale, say around 100°F (38°C).

Storage Containers

I like containers that are aesthetically pleasing, but it's more important to select ones that are appropriate for the product, such as a spritzer bottle for sprays, a 10 ml roller-ball applicator for a roll-on remedy, or an unbreakable PET plastic squeeze bottle for herbal oils.

Many retailers carry suitable containers. Check with arts and crafts suppliers, hardware stores, home goods stores, herb shops, larger health food stores, and grocers that cater to healthy lifestyles. If you can't find what you want locally, search the Internet. As always, buying in bulk saves money. Sharing the container order with a friend or two saves money as well. I generally purchase containers by the dozen from mail-order bottle companies and a few of my favorite mail-order herb shops (see Resources, page 229).

BOTTLES. You'll need a variety to hold all your liquid creations:

+ 5 ml bottles (dark glass, with orifice reducer dropper inserts) hold up to 100 drops of essential oil. They're convenient for small amounts of your favorite diffuser blends.

+ 10 ml roll-on applicator bottles (glass) are perfect for oil- or vodka-based spot-treatment blends, lip glosses, or your favorite relaxing or energizing aromas.

+ Boston rounds (glass or plastic) are available in many sizes with screw-on, pump, dropper top, or spritzer tops. Use these narrow-neck bottles to store products such as base oils, infused oils, oil blends, liniments, mouthwash, room sprays, facial mists, deodorants, and breath sprays.

CANNING JARS. These clear glass jars come in a variety of sizes and are suitable for storing such things as dried herbs, powdered clay, tooth powder, Epsom salt, beeswax pastilles, cocoa butter wafers, liniments, and infused herbal oils (when kept away from light) and for making solar-infused oils.

CREAM JARS. In a range of sizes, and available in glass or plastic, they are the containers of choice for storing balms, salves, homemade toothpastes or tooth powders, and body scrubs. The amber, green, and cobalt blue glass jars are my favorites due to their aesthetic appeal, heft, and classic apothecary look. Some retailers sell "double wall" plastic jars, and though not made from PET or HDPE plastic, they are safe for the products just mentioned.

INHALER STICKS. Also called nasal inhaler blanks, aroma sticks, or (my favorite) sniffy sticks, these portable personal inhalation tubes allow you to conveniently take your favorite essential oil blend with you anywhere. Just saturate the cotton wick with approximately 14 to 24 drops of essential oil, depending on the formula, insert it into the base tube, and add the bottom plug. I prefer the aluminum sticks with an interior glass tube to the plastic ones, as they are easily rechargeable and durable. The less expensive, disposable plastic versions are neither.

TINS. Having a round, flat shape, these metal containers are available in many sizes. They should be seamless, with a safe-edge body and a plain, tight-fitting push-on lid. The smaller tins are ideal for lip balms, for travel-size portions of remedial salves and balms, and for stacking in first-aid kits. I like to use the larger tins to store batches of tooth powder, body powder, and bath salt blends and single dry ingredients such as Epsom salt, powdered kaolin clay, baking soda, dried herbs, beeswax pastilles, and cocoa butter wafers.

ZIPLOCK FREEZER BAGS. Dried herbs are best stored in tightly sealed jars or tins, but ziplock freezer bags are a reasonable and inexpensive alternative, and they're fine for baking soda, kaolin clay, Epsom salt, beeswax pastilles, cocoa butter wafers, and other dry ingredients. If you do use them to store herbs, keep them in a very dry, cool, dark place and use the herbs within a year. Note: The slide-lock freezer bags are *not* airtight; use the double-zipper style instead.

Label, Label, Label!

Always label your creations with the ingredients, instructions for use, the date it was made, the expiration date, and the words "For External Use Only," if applicable. Any type of label is fine, but because the containers may get handled by wet or oily hands, protect labels with clear shipping tape or laminating sheets.

If you find that you enjoy making essential oil remedies for friends and family, then design a label that is uniquely yours by using a computer label program, or hand-print your labels, or perhaps find a local print shop that can help you with a custom design. Just make sure your ink is water- and smear-proof!

Keep It Clean

"Cleanliness is next to godliness" — there's a good reason why I say this in all of my books. I'm a stickler about proper sanitation. Prior to use, every implement, piece of equipment, and storage container should be run through the dishwasher or washed in very hot soapy water and allowed to air-dry, upside down, on a rack. You don't want to introduce bacteria into your newly made products by using dirty tools or storage containers (or dirty hands)! Thoroughly clean and dry all your utensils after using them as well.

Glass versus Plastic

Generally speaking, dark glass (amber, cobalt blue, or dark green) is the best option when it comes to storing your home remedies, as the tint helps preserve the volatile properties contained within the botanical liquids against the damaging effects of bright light. Plus, glass won't react with the chemical constituents in the essential oils or herbs. If you are decanting pure undiluted essential oils from larger to smaller containers, dark glass is a must, and concentrations of essential oils should *always* be stored in glass. I like glass and love its heft, look, and feel.

However, in some cases it's impossible, impractical, or downright inconvenient to use glass for your natural concoctions, such as when you are traveling, if you have small children and pets, or if you are storing containers in the shower or carrying them with you in a purse or backpack. Plastic can be a viable option, but you have to use the right type and essential oils *must always be diluted* before being stored in plastic containers because they can degrade it over time, leaching the plastic's chemicals into the product. Here's what to look for:

PET plastic: Polyethylene terephthalate is safe, nontoxic, strong, lightweight, flexible, and recyclable. It is available in standard clear or clear cobalt blue, green, or amber bottles and jars, plus some solid colors. The #1 recycle symbol appears on the bottom of the container. When I must use a plastic container, PET plastic is my favorite.

HDPE plastic: High-density polyethylene is safe, nontoxic, super-strong, lightweight, flexible, recyclable, impact resistant, weather-resistant, and long-lasting. It is available in bottles and jars, typically opaque, but also in a few solid colors. The #2 recycle symbol appears on the bottom of the container.

APPENDIX: Making Herb-Infused Oils

There are several methods for making an infused oil, but since this is a beginner's guide, let's keep things nice and simple. I'll teach you my two favorite methods: the solar, or sun, infusion method and the stovetop method. Both methods work well, are easy to follow, and ensure a good end product. But first, I need to mention a few important points before we get into the meat of preparation.

Use Quality Ingredients

The quality of the herbs you use is as important to herbalism as the purity of essential oils is to aromatherapy. While growing your own organic herbs is ideal, I realize that many people must purchase herbs in dried form from herb shops or Internet sources. You can determine whether a dried herb is of good quality by smelling, seeing, and tasting it. Dried herbs should not be lifeless with minimal scent; they should be colorful (or at least a muted version of the fresh herb), vibrant, and fragrant.

Look for herbs that were responsibly and sustainably harvested in the wild or organically grown. Purchasing directly from the wildcrafter (one who picks and processes wild herbs) or the grower, perhaps at a farmers' market or through a community-supported agriculture (CSA) farm, where you can inquire about growing methods, is an excellent alternative to growing and drying your own herbs.

I highly recommend using organic oils. Oil derived from beans, nuts, seeds, fruits, and grains — that is, vegetable oil — is a good extractive medium not only for the fat-soluble constituents of plants, but also for agricultural chemicals, including herbicides and pesticides. Organic extra-virgin olive oil is my favorite choice for making herbal infused oils, as it is medicinal in its own right, although other minimally processed superior-quality base oils such as jojoba, sesame, or almond may also be used.

Use Promptly . . .

Unlike dried herbs, which can be stored in airtight containers at room temperature for a year or longer, wilted herbs are still relatively fresh and cannot be stored for any length of time. They must be picked, prepped, and wilted within a few days prior to when you intend to make a given recipe.

When you make an infused oil from fresh herbs, you will need to wilt (partially dry) the herbs first. The process removes sufficient moisture from the plant material to inhibit mold and bacterial growth — and the potential for a layer of watery sludge to form on the bottom of the storage jar — without affecting the healing properties.

I rarely have a problem with excess moisture or mold when I make an infused oil using freshly wilted herbs, but if I do, it's because I didn't wilt the herb long enough or because my jar or lid was damp. I recommend considerably longer wilting times than those recommended by most herbalists. You're more likely to produce a superb healing oil on your first try, without having to toss the entire batch because something went awry. That's a waste of time, money, oil, and herbs!

The process of wilting is simple. Let's take calendula blossoms as an example. Pick approximately double the amount of blossoms as the recipe calls for to allow for shrinkage, making sure to include the entire flower head, not just the petals. Flowers with petals shrink considerably when wilted, while tight lavender buds and chamomile flowers don't as much. You'll learn through trial and error how much fresh material to pick; it's not an exact science.

Snip the calendula blossoms after the morning dew has dried, but before the sun gets too warm. These are thick, sticky flowers, so gently tear or shred them a bit by hand to expose more surface area so that they wilt more evenly. Spread the flowers and any bits of attached greenery on a clean screen, pillowcase, or length of lint-free cloth (a long strip of paper towels will do) in a warm, relatively still location that is mostly shady and is protected from flies and wafting animal dander and dust.

I usually wilt my herbs on a table or shelf in my study or in the backseat of my hot car on sunny summer and early autumn days — away from my curious cats. Utilizing my car's concentrated heat, I've discovered, is a quick way to obtain nearly dry herbs in a matter of days!

Allow the flowers to wilt for 72 hours. (Calendula flowers take longer to thoroughly wilt than many other herbs, as they contain more moisture. Most flowers take between 24 and 48 hours.) If the humidity is very high, add another 24 hours. You should notice a distinct change in texture, from firm and fresh to limp and soft, or even a bit on the leathery side, especially if the temperature is over 90°F (32°C) and the humidity quite low. The size of the flower will diminish as the water evaporates out of the plant material. The amount of shrinkage depends on the temperature and level of humidity; the warmer and drier, the greater the reduction in herb size.

Solar Infusion Method

People have been successfully harnessing the sun's energy to extract oil from herbal constituents for thousands of years. This is my preferred method. It may not be the quickest, but I feel that by allowing universal energy systems to create the healing potion according to their timetable, not mine, I receive a super-charged medicine, a true gift from Mother Nature. She provides the medicinal plants and the solar and lunar energy. I simply join them together and reap the benefits of what I call "plant spirit vibrational earth medicine in a bottle."

1. Place 2 cups of dried herbs or 4 cups of wilted plant matter into a clean, dry, wide-mouthed 1-quart jar. Cut or tear wilted herbs into small pieces.

2. Pour 3 to 4 cups of base oil over the plant matter, until the oil comes to within 1 inch of the top of the jar. The dried herb may pack in the bottom and the wilted herb matter will settle with the weight of the oil, so don't worry if it looks as though you don't have enough plant matter in the jar. Gently stir to remove air bubbles and make sure that all the plant matter is submerged.

3. Place a piece of plastic wrap over the mouth of the jar (to prevent the metal lid from coming into contact with the herbs) and tightly screw on the lid.

Shake the jar several times to blend the herbs and oil thoroughly. Place the jar in a warm, sunny location, such as a south-facing windowsill, or outside if the daytime temperatures are consistently over 80°F (27°C). Allow the herb to infuse for 1 month, shaking the jar every day for 30 seconds or so. Ideally, I begin my solar infusions on the first day of the full moon and strain them out on the next full moon.

4. After 1 month, carefully strain the oil through a fine-mesh strainer lined with a fine filter such as muslin cloth or, preferably, a paper coffee filter, then strain again if necessary to remove all herb debris. Squeeze the herbs to extract as much of the precious oil as possible. Discard the spent herbs. Add 7 capsules of 400 IU vitamin E oil as a preservative and stir to blend. The yield will be 2½ to 3½ cups of infused oil, depending on whether you used dried or fresh herbs and how much oil you added.

5. Pour the infused oil into dark glass bottles or jars. Label and date your product and store in a cool, dark cabinet; use within 1 year.

Stovetop Infusion Method

Another way to infuse oils uses direct heat on the stovetop, and it allows you to infuse an oil in hours rather than weeks.

1. Place 1½ cups of dried herbs or 3 cups of wilted plant matter in the top part of a medium-size double boiler or in a saucepan. Cut or tear wilted herbs into small pieces. I *strongly* recommend using a double boiler instead of a regular saucepan, as the oil can quickly overheat. You don't want to fry your herbs or burn your oil, and either can happen in the blink of an eye if you're not using a double boiler. I've learned the hard way. It's easy to get distracted!

2. Pour 3 cups of base oil over the herbs and stir thoroughly to blend. Bring the mixture to just shy of a simmer (preferably between 100° and 125°F/38° and 52°C). *Do not* let the oil actually simmer — it will degrade the quality of your infused oil. *Do not* put the lid on the saucepan or the double boiler.

3. Allow the herb to infuse in the oil for 4 hours or so, until the oil takes on the color and scent of the herb. (Note that St. John's Wort–infused oil will turn a vibrant red and not yellow like the flowers.) Every 30 minutes, give the herbs a quick stir and also check the temperature with a candy or yogurt thermometer, adjusting the heat accordingly. If you're using a double boiler, add more water to the bottom pot as necessary, so it doesn't dry out.

4. After 4 hours, remove the pan from the heat and allow the oil to cool for 15 minutes. While the oil is still warm, carefully strain it through a fine-mesh strainer lined with a fine filter such as muslin cloth or, preferably, a paper coffee filter, then strain again if necessary to remove all herb debris. Squeeze the herbs to extract as much of the precious oil as possible. Discard the spent herbs. Add 7 capsules of 400 IU vitamin E oil as a preservative and stir to blend. The yield will be approximately 2½ to 2¾ cups of infused oil.

5. Pour the infused oil into dark glass bottles or jars. Label and date your product and store in a cool, dark cabinet; use within 1 year.

Resources
Suppliers

The Ananda Apothecary
888-758-6360
www.anandaapothecary.com
Therapeutic-grade essential oils and blends, hydrosols, aromatherapy supplies, base oils, bottles, essential oil diffusers, and books

AromaTherapeutix
800-308-6284
www.aromatherapeutix.com
Huge variety of essential oils and oil blends, bottles, soaps, herbal body and health care products, essential oil diffusers, and more

Aromatics International
406-273-9833
www.aromatics.com
Organic and wildcrafted essential oils and oil blends, hydrosols, base oils, essential oil accessories, and packaging

Aura Cacia
Frontier Natural Products Co-op
800-437-3301
www.auracacia.com
Essential oils, base oils, and natural skin and body care products

dōTERRA
Stephanie Tourles, Wellness Advocate
Professional Aromatherapist/Licensed Esthetician/Certified Foot & Hand Reflexologist
https://mydoterra.com/stephanietourles

Superior-quality therapeutic-grade essential oils and blends, aromatherapy kits, nutritional supplements, and body care products. I personally use these in my holistic skin care and reflexology practice – with amazing results!

Eden Botanicals
707-509-0041
www.edenbotanicals.com
Specializing in wholesale essential oils, CO_2 extracts, and absolutes for aromatherapy, natural perfumery, and body and facial care. Superior quality.

Frontier Natural Products Co-op
800-669-3275
www.frontiercoop.com
Large inventory of essential oils, base oils, organic herbs, spices, teas, dried foods, cosmetic clays, beeswax, and natural body care products

Healthy Harvest
www.healthyharvests.com
Best olive oils ever, plus aromatherapeutic facial oil blends formulated by Stephanie Tourles

Jean's Greens
518-479-0471
www.jeansgreens.com
A wide range of wonderful herb products, teas, loose herbs and spices, essential oils, beeswax, butters, cosmetic clays, books, and more

Mountain Rose Herbs
800-879-3337
www.mountainroseherbs.com
Organic bulk herbs, spices, teas, essential and base oils, packaging supplies, herbal health aids, natural personal care products, and more

Original Swiss Aromatics
415-479-9120
www.originalswissaromatics.com
Superior-quality, authentic organic and wildcrafted essential oils, plus facial, massage, and body care oils, hydrosols, and natural perfumes

Simplers Botanicals
NutraMarks
800-229-2512
www.simplers.com
Superior-quality therapeutic-grade organic and wildcrafted essential oils, hydrosols, natural perfume oils, infused herbal oils, herbal extracts, and more

Specialty Bottle
206-382-1100
www.specialtybottle.com
Glass and plastic bottles, jars, and tins of every size imaginable

SKS Bottle & Packaging, Inc.
518-880-6980
www.sks-bottle.com
Glass and plastic bottles, jars, and tins of all sizes

Stillpoint Aromatics
928-301-8699
www.stillpointaromatics.com
Exceptional-quality essential oils, aromatherapy kits, hydrosols, flower essences, base oils, infused oils, books, and more

Aromatherapy Education & Associations

Alliance of International Aromatherapists
877-531-6377
www.alliance-aromatherapists.org
A member-based nonprofit organization providing education using scientific research and traditional information to promote the responsible use of aromatherapy. They serve the public, researchers, educators, health care professionals, industry, and the media. AIA maintains a list of approved aromatherapy schools and practitioners.

American College of Healthcare Sciences
800-487-8839
www.achs.edu
An accredited online and on-campus college offering holistic health and aromatherapy education

Aromahead Institute
727-469-3134
www.aromahead.com
Online aromatherapy certification programs, webinars on aromatherapy, body, and healthcare subjects, continuing education credits, books, and more

Atlantic Institute of Aromatherapy
813-265-2222
www.atlanticinstitute.com
Offers hands-on classes for beginners and seasoned practitioners alike, home-study course, and educational products

Canadian Federation of Aromatherapists
519-746-1594
www.cfacanada.com

International Federation of Professional Aromatherapists
+44-0-145-563-7987
www.ifparoma.org

Tisserand Institute
www.tisserandinstitute.org
Owned by Robert Tisserand, one of the world's leading aromatherapy experts. Mr. Tisserand serves as an industry consultant, online educator, and live presenter and is the author of several highly regarded essential oil books. His institute synthesizes and translates new research and scientific findings into comprehensive and meaningful educational material on the benefits of safe use of essential oils. Excellent webinars available – enthusiastically recommended!

National Association for Holistic Aromatherapy
919-894-0298
www.naha.org

A nonprofit educational organization dedicated to enhancing public awareness, perception, and knowledge of the benefits of true aromatherapy and its safe and effective application in everyday life. NAHA maintains a listing of approved aromatherapy schools and practitioners, plus offers books, a calendar of events, and an online journal to members.

Pacific Institute of Aromatherapy
415-479-9120
www.pacificinstituteofaromatherapy.com
In-depth correspondence courses in French-style aromatherapy. Highly recommended!

School of Holistic Aromatherapy
www.holisticaroma.co.uk

Stillpoint Studies
Stillpoint Aromatics
928-301-7544
www.stillpointstudies.com
Excellent certification programs and workshops in aromatherapy, from beginner to advanced. Hands-on training in a classroom setting.

West Coast Institute of Aromatherapy
604-736-7476
www.westcoastaromatherapy.com
Offers home-study aromatherapy correspondence courses, from beginner to the clinical aromatherapist level, plus other related workshops

Recommended Reading

This list contains many of the resources for this book as well as selections from my personal library. If you're interested in the study of essential oils, aromatherapy, and natural self-care, you'll find them all quite educational and enlightening.

Clarke, Sue. *Essential Chemistry for Aromatherapy.* 2nd ed. Elsevier Health Sciences, 2008.

Cooksley, Valerie Gennari, R.N. *Aromatherapy: Soothing Remedies to Restore, Rejuvenate, and Heal.* Prentice Hall, 2002.

Curtis, Susan. *Essential Oils.* Revised & updated ed. Winter Press, 2014.

Gladstar, Rosemary. *Rosemary Gladstar's Medicinal Herbs: A Beginner's Guide.* Storey Publishing, 2012.

Green, Mindy, Kathi Keville. *Aromatherapy: A Complete Guide to The Healing Art.* 2nd ed. Crossing Press, 2009.

Lawless, Julia. *The Illustrated Encyclopedia of Essential Oils: The Complete Guide to the Use of Oils in Aromatherapy and Herbalism.* Element Books, 1995.

Miller, Bryan, D.C., and Light Miller, N.D. *Ayurveda & Aromatherapy: The Earth Essential Guide to Ancient Wisdom and Modern Healing.* Lotus Press, 1995.

Ody, Penelope. *The Complete Medicinal Herbal.* Dorling Kindersley, 1993.

Penoel, Daniel, M.D., and Rose-Marie Penoel. *Life Helping Life: Unleash Your Mind/Body Potential with Essential Oils.* Essentia Publishing, 2000.

Purchon, Nerys, and Lora Cantele. *The Complete Aromatherapy & Essential Oils Handbook for Everyday Wellness.* Robert Rose, Inc., 2014.

Schnaubelt, Kurt, Ph.D. *Advanced Aromatherapy: The Science of Essential Oil Therapy.* Healing Arts Press, 1998

Schnaubelt, Kurt, Ph.D. *Medical Aromatherapy: Healing with Essential Oils.* Frog, Ltd., 1999.

Schnaubelt, Kurt, Ph.D. *The Healing Intelligence of Essential Oils: The Science of Advanced Aromatherapy.* Healing Arts Press, 2011.

Tisserand, Robert B. *The Art of Aromatherapy: The Healing and Beautifying Properties of the Essential Oils of Flowers and Herbs.* Healing Arts Press, 1977.

Tisserand, Robert, and Rodney Young, Ph.D. *Essential Oil Safety: A Guide for Health Care Professionals.* 2nd ed. Churchill Livingstone, 2014.

Tourles, Stephanie. *Organic Body Care Recipes: 175 Homemade Herbal Formulas for Glowing Skin & a Vibrant Self.* Storey Publishing, 2007.

Tourles, Stephanie. *Hands-On Healing Remedies: 150 Recipes for Herbal Balms, Salves, Oils, Liniments & Other Topical Therapies.* Storey Publishing, 2012.

Walters, Clare. *Aromatherapy: An Illustrated Guide.* Element Books, 1998.

Worwood, Valerie Ann. *The Complete Book of Essential Oils and Aromatherapy.* 25th Anniversary ed. New World Library, 2016.

Acknowledgments

I am indebted to the following people, who, over the past five decades, have contributed greatly to my knowledge and appreciation of the natural world — guiding me in this lifelong journey and exploration of healing herbs and essential oils: My mother, Brenda Anchors, who taught me to garden organically, build a compost pile, and plant amazingly beautiful flower boxes; the late Earl C. Ashe, my grandfather and first herb teacher, who showed me how to use plants for medicine and skin care; the late Phenie S. Ashe, my grandmother, who possessed the greenest thumb on Earth and enthusiastically suggested that I both talk to and touch my plants, thus encouraging them to produce bounteously.

Also to Robin Lander, herbalist, aromatherapist, and formulator and sourcing specialist at Simplers Botanicals, for answering more than a few questions and sending me many samples to experiment with and share with my students; Rosemary Gladstar, Candis Cantin, and Deb Soule, my favorite instructors with whom I've studied varying traditions of herbal wisdom; and the following group of consultants, educators, and authors in the fields of aromatherapy and herbalism who continue to work tirelessly to promote planetary and personal healing through the use of essential oils and herbs — you have inspired and enlightened: Robert Tisserand, Maggie Tisserand, Sue Clarke, Jeanne Rose, Light Miller, N.D., Bryan Miller, D.C., Valerie Cooksley, R.N., Daniel Pénoël, M.D., Julia Lawless, Kurt Schnaubelt, Ph.D., Marcel Lavabre, Kathi Keville, Mindy Green, Lora Cantele, and Valerie Ann Worwood.

Many thanks to my family, friends, and clients who graciously volunteered to be live subjects on whom I could test my aromatherapeutic formulations and receive much valued feedback. Your opinions and suggestions were greatly appreciated! Special gratitude flows to Deborah Balmuth, Storey's publisher, for her continued faith in my abilities and for granting me the opportunity to share the aromatic realm of the herb world with you, my dear readers. And to my longtime editor, Lisa Hiley — thanks for always being a pleasure to work with!

Praise be to the good Lord above for creating the plants — they are our blessed gifts for sustenance, comfort, and medicine.

Index

Expand Your Natural Self-Care Education with More Books by Stephanie L. Tourles

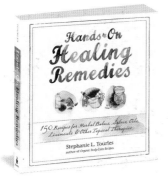

Fill your medicine cabinet with all-natural, topical handmade herbal remedies. More than 100 recipes for liniments, balms, and essential oil blends will help you treat a range of ailments, from arthritis to warts.

Protect yourself from mosquitoes, ticks, and other biting insects without relying on chemicals. These 75 all-natural recipes for sprays, balms, body oils, and tinctures — plus herbal pet shampoos, flea collars, and powders — are safe for your body, pets, and home.

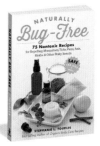

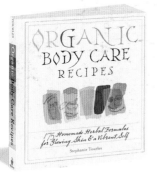

Maintain radiantly healthy and beautiful skin, hair, and body with these fun and simple recipes for creams, scrubs, toners, and much more. This wide range of beauty formulas will pamper you from head to toe with nourishing, natural ingredients.